Allergy

YOUR QUESTIONS ANSWERED

Commissioning and Project Development: Fiona Conn
Project Management: Frances Affleck
Design Direction: George Ajayi

Allergy

YOUR QUESTIONS ANSWERED

Helen E Smith
DM FFPHM MRCGP
Reader in Primary Care, School of Medicine,
University of Southampton, UK

Anthony J Frew
MA MD FRCP
Professor of Allergy and Respiratory Medicine,
School of Medicine, University of Southampton, UK

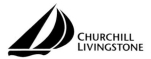

CHURCHILL
LIVINGSTONE

EDINBURGH LONDON NEW YORK OXFORD PHILADELPHIA ST LOUIS SYDNEY TORONTO 2003

CHURCHILL LIVINGSTONE
An imprint of Elsevier Science Limited

First published 2003

ISBN 0 4430 7291 4

British Library Cataloguing in Publication Data
A catalogue record for this book is available from the British Library

Library of Congress Cataloging in Publication Data
A catalog record for this book is available from the Library of Congress

Notice
Medical knowledge is constantly changing. Standard safety precautions must be followed,
but as new research and clinical experience broaden our knowledge, changes in treatment
and drug therapy may become necessary or appropriate. Readers are advised to check the
most current product information provided by the manufacturer of each drug to be
administered to verify the recommended dose, the method and duration of administration,
and contraindications. It is the responsibility of the practitioner, relying on experience and
knowledge of the patient, to determine dosages and the best treatment for each individual
patient. Neither the Publisher nor the authors assume any liability for any injury and/or
damage to persons or property arising from this publication.
The Publisher

ELSEVIER
SCIENCE
your source for books,
journals and multimedia
in the health sciences
www.elsevierhealth.com

The
publisher's
policy is to use
paper manufactured
from sustainable forests

Printed in China

Contents

Preface

Allergic conditions are extremely common and have increased considerably in frequency in the past 30–40 years. Fortunately, most people with allergic conditions have relatively mild disease and are able to manage their symptoms themselves, sometimes with advice from their local pharmacist or their friends. However, some allergies are more serious and worrying, leading patients to seek advice from primary care teams. At the other end of the spectrum, a few patients have life-threatening allergies such as anaphylactic reactions to food and drugs that may require emergency treatment in A&E departments or admission to hospital. At the same time, many people believe that a wide range of other symptoms are due to allergy, when in fact there is little evidence that allergy is really responsible.

Allergy does not feature very large in medical training: some medical schools have a couple of lectures on the subject, and others have none at all. As a result, many doctors feel that they are inadequately informed to answer patients' questions on allergic disease. This book seeks to fill that gap by providing answers to a wide range of questions that have been raised by patients and doctors. Many of the questions posed here are based on referral letters to our Allergy Clinics, and others arise from discussions with patients. We hope that, by offering practical and down-to-earth advice for patients and doctors alike, we may go a little way to improve the welfare of the many patients with allergic conditions who are seeking answers to their legitimate questions, and are not always sure where they should turn.

HS
AF

How to use this book

The *Your Questions Answered* series aims to meet the information needs of GPs and other primary care professionals who care for patients with chronic conditions. It is designed to help them work with patients and their families, providing effective, evidence-based care and management.

The books are in an accessible question and answer format, with detailed contents lists at the beginning of every chapter and a complete index to help find specific information.

ICONS

Icons are used in the book to identify particular types of information:

 highlights important information

 highlights side-effect information.

PATIENT QUESTIONS

At the end of relevant chapters there are sections of frequently asked patient questions, with easy-to-understand answers aimed at the non-medical reader. These questions are also listed at the end of the book.

Allergy and allergens

INTRODUCTION

1.1 What is allergy?

The word allergy was coined in the 19th century from the Greek words 'allon argon' and means to react differently. Allergic people respond differently to certain substances in that they develop hypersensitivity reactions to various foods, drugs, inhaled particles, etc., leading to symptoms and illness.

1.2 What is atopy?

Atopy is not an illness but rather the characteristic which makes people more likely to develop an allergic disorder. Atopic people inherit a predisposition to develop allergy and may or may not go on to have symptoms. Atopic people have an overdeveloped ability to develop sensitizing antibodies, known as immunoglobulin E (IgE) to otherwise harmless foreign materials like pollens, animal dander, foods, etc. This tendency is genetically controlled (at least five distinct genetic areas have been implicated). Whether the atopic tendency goes on to be expressed as symptoms depends on a range of environmental factors. The relationship between atopy and allergy is thus a good example of gene–environment interaction.

1.3 Where does the word atopy come from?

Like allergy, atopy is derived from Greek. 'Topos' means a place and 'atopos' means out of place.

1.4 How common is allergy?

The proportion of people with allergic sensitization varies widely from country to country (*Fig. 1.1*), with higher rates in developed countries, especially the UK, US and old commonwealth (Australia and New Zealand being the worst affected).

1.5 What medical conditions are caused by allergy? (See *Table 1.1*)

The commonest allergic condition is allergic rhinitis. Asthma, anaphylaxis, urticaria and eczema can all be due to allergy, although the proportion of cases that involve allergy varies widely from condition to condition. Some doctors and healthcare advisors believe that a wider range of conditions can be caused by allergies, or by exposure to foods and environmental chemicals. (See section on alternative/complementary medicine and allergy, pp. 163–174.)

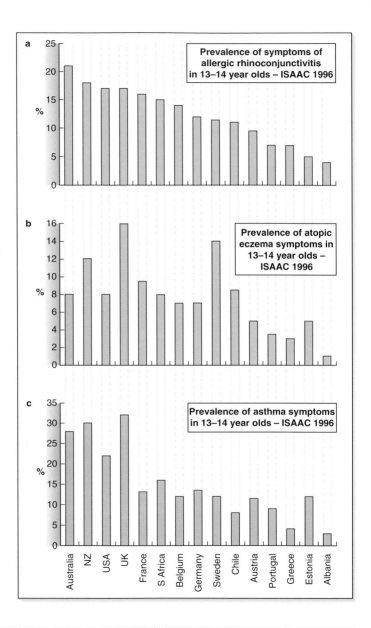

Fig 1.1 Frequency of allergy in different countries. Data based on Beasley R et al. 1998 Worldwide variation in prevalence of symptoms of asthma, allergic rhinoconjunctivitis and atopic eczema: ISAAC The Lancet 351: 1225–1232.

TABLE 1.1 Relative role of allergy in different conditions	
Conjunctivitis	Some
Seasonal rhinitis	Almost all
Perennial rhinitis	50:50
Childhood asthma	Predisposing
Adult asthma	Less important
Urticaria/angioedema	<10%
Anaphylaxis	Most

1.6 Is food allergy a defined condition?

Strictly speaking, food allergy is a trigger for allergic symptoms rather than a condition in its own right. Most patients with food allergy will have symptoms in and around the mouth shortly after eating the food to which they are allergic. Some will have urticaria and/or angioedema; a few will experience generalized anaphylactic reactions. Food can trigger attacks of asthma, rhinitis or eczema, usually as part of a more generalized reaction, but is a relatively unusual cause of isolated allergic symptoms.

1.7 Is allergy a growing problem or is it just a diagnostic fashion?

Allergies have been recognized for hundreds of years. As early as 1570 a man's allergy to cats was recognized when he became agitated, broke into a sweat and developed blisters on entering a room with a cat. However, hay fever and asthma were pretty rare until the end of the 19th century. The recent escalation in allergic problems arises for a number of reasons:

- Improved knowledge (some previously unexplained conditions are now recognized as allergic in origin).
- Increased recognition and labelling of allergic conditions as such.
- Real increase (largely post-1960, as clearly shown in Germany, comparing those born in West and East Germany, where there is no difference in rates of allergy in the two regions in those born before 1960, but then a widening gap in rates of allergy between the two parts in those born afterwards, see p. 29)
- Increased use of medical services. (Within the UK, there has been a dramatic rise in the number of people using medical services for allergic conditions, which is several times steeper than the rise in the rates of sensitization.)

Thus, we are looking at a combination of increased rates of sensitization, increased likelihood of sensitization progressing to disease, increased recognition of allergy and increased use of medical services.

1.8   What is an allergen?

An allergen is a protein or chemical that is capable of causing sensitization and subsequent allergic sensitivity on re-exposure. Everyone's immune system can recognize the allergen, but only those with an atopic tendency will be able to make sensitizing antibodies to it.

1.9   What are the commonest allergens in the UK?

In rank order, house dust mites (*Fig. 1.2a*), grass pollen, cat dander (*Fig. 1.2b*) and tree pollen are the commonest inhalant allergens. Common food allergens include shellfish, peanuts, tree nuts, strawberries, with cow's

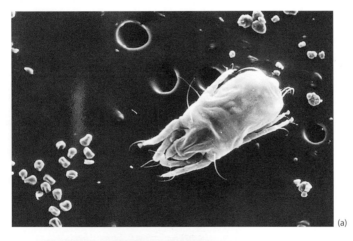

(a)

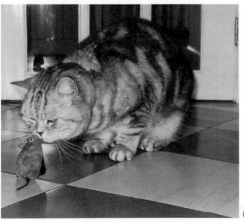

(b)

◀ **Fig 1.2** a) House dust mites: Dermatophagoids pteronyssinus photographed with a scanning electron microscope. From Roitt I, Brostoff J, Male D (eds) 2001 Immunology. Edinburgh: Mosby, with permission b) Cats (Felix domesticus) produce potent allergens in their sebaceous gland secretions. Once dried, it comes off the skin and hair and is then distributed widely in the house. From Crockett A 2003 Asthma: Your Questions Answered. Edinburgh: Churchill Livingstone, with permission.

milk and egg particularly troublesome in early childhood. Other relevant allergens include mould spores, insect venom, latex and various chemicals and drugs. (See section on occupational allergens, pp. 143–149)

1.10   What makes an allergen an allergen?

There are two distinct elements: firstly, the allergenic protein has to be presented in a way that will allow it to reach the mucous membranes; secondly, it must have properties that fool the body into making IgE directed against the allergenic protein. Plants that rely on wind pollination are much more likely to cause problems than plants which use insects for pollination. A good guide is that plants that rely on insects have gaudy flowers and nectar to attract the insects. Their pollens are sticky and heavy, so that they will stick to the insect and be carried to the next flower. Consequently, these pollens are not represented to any significant extent in ambient air and are not available to be inhaled. People with allergies may be affected by the scent of the flower but will not generally be sensitized to the plant. In contrast, wind-pollinated plants have small inconspicuous flowers and do not make nectar. Some pollens are the right size to be inhaled; others are too big, but they may fragment into smaller particles or the proteins may be carried into the lungs by diesel exhaust particles or other respirable particles.

Many allergens are enzymes which can digest other proteins. For example, house dust mite allergens are the digestive proteins that house dust mites secrete to digest those particles of human skin off which they live. They chew up the skin and then deposit small faecal pellets which consist of a small piece of human skin covered in their digestive enzymes. The skin degrades inside the pellet, and later on the mite can come back and eat the particle which is now digestible. The enzymes are harmless to us, and would not cause any problem if the faecal pellets were larger, but they happen to be just the right size to be inhaled.

Pollen and cat dander allergens can also be enzymes, and it has been suggested that the body thinks it is under attack by something that is trying to digest its way into the body. This is similar to what happens with intestinal worms, and it is noteworthy that anyone with intestinal worms will make very strong IgE responses against the worm proteins. The ability to make such responses could have conferred an evolutionary advantage in the past, but now it just makes you prone to allergic reactions against otherwise harmless proteins.

Allergenic chemicals generally bind to human proteins to form complex targets for the immune system. Certain types of chemical seem to be more capable of doing this than others. Researchers are now trying to use the structure of chemicals to predict whether they are likely to be allergenic.

Other researchers believe that protein allergens may have similar 3D structures, and this may encourage the immune system to make a stereotyped response. Understanding more about this would help us to assess the risks of new material being allergenic, but the first principle in industry and domestic settings is to minimize unnecessary exposure to potentially hazardous materials, especially in aerosol form.

1.11   What other factors are involved in allergy?

The single biggest risk factor for becoming sensitized to new proteins and chemicals is to be allergic to other things already. In part this reflects the possession of the genetic risk factors for making IgE responses, but it may also be driven by having an inflamed nasal and airways mucosa. Early treatment of children with house dust mite allergy by immunotherapy (and possibly also with antihistamines) seems to reduce the risk of them becoming sensitized to other agents, such as grass pollen and cat dander, as they get older.

Among children of atopic parents, the risk of sensitization to foods is increased by the early introduction of solid foods (especially eggs and cow's milk).

Smoking is also implicated as a risk factor for allergy. Children whose parents smoke show increased rates of allergic sensitization, while adults who smoke are at increased risk of occupational allergic asthma if they are exposed to allergens such as acid anhydrides and platinum.

1.12   Are microbes allergenic in humans?

The relationship between infection and allergy is complex. In some parts of Europe, doctors and patients believe that allergy to bacteria is a real problem and they vaccinate allergic children against bacteria; however, this is not generally accepted in the West.

Normal gut bacteria are important in shaping the immune system in the first few weeks after birth. Changes in the gut bacterial flora may have been important in allowing the current generation of children to develop allergies, but these allergies are directed against pollens, mites and animal dander, not against the bacteria. Most bacteria induce Th1-type immune responses which are more likely to be protective than allergenic. Viruses generally trigger cell-mediated responses that kill infected cells, and antibody responses that protect the patient from future infection. One particular virus (respiratory syncytial virus [RSV]) is unusual in that it triggers a Th2-type immune response to some of its proteins. *Staphylococcus aureus* may be important in exacerbations of eczema, through production of T cell activating enterotoxins (see Chapter 8).

DIAGNOSIS

1.13 How can one confirm a diagnosis of allergy?

The most important step is to take a good history (*Box 1.1*), identifying the patient's clinical problems, and then exploring possible trigger factors for their symptoms. Wherever possible, the list of symptoms should be kept separate from issues of causation. Clinical examination is not particularly helpful in assessing whether symptoms are allergic in origin, but should be used to exclude other conditions. Having clarified the history, the extent and severity of the allergic sensitization can be assessed by skin tests, blood tests or direct challenges.

1.14 Is skin prick testing safe?

Yes. Skin prick testing involves placing a drop of an allergen extract on to the skin and then introducing a small amount into the epidermis with a calibrated lancet (*Fig. 1.3*). If the patient is allergic to the extract, they will react to the test substance by releasing histamine from local mast cells, which shows up as a small weal, like a nettle sting. This is a simple procedure and, when performed by a trained person and interpreted in conjunction with an allergy history, provides an accurate assessment of allergic disorders. Skin prick testing is very safe in patients whose problem is rhinitis or asthma, providing that standardized allergen extracts are used. Caution should be exercised when testing patients with a history of anaphylaxis, or when using non-commercial extracts.

BOX 1.1 Key elements of an allergy history

Clinical problem

Onset and course
- Seasonality/persistence
- Aggravating factors
- Sleep pattern
- Personal history of atopy in childhood
- Sensitivities — known and suspected
- Family history of allergic disorders
- Home environment (age, period of residence, carpets, smoking, pets)
- Work and workplace
- Medication (current and previous)

General history
- Occupation; activity; limitations; smoking (self and other household members)

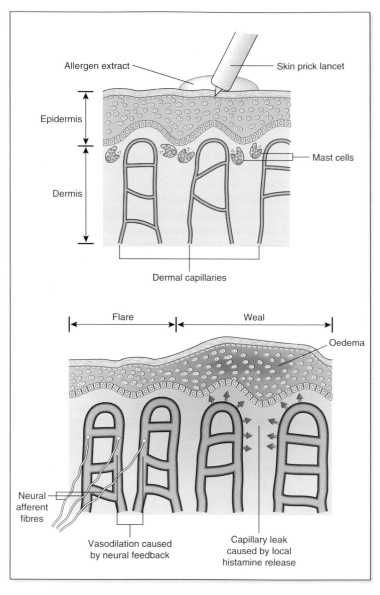

Allergen extract

Skin prick lancet

Epidermis

Mast cells

Dermis

Dermal capillaries

Flare

Weal

Oedema

Neural afferent fibres

Vasodilation caused by neural feedback

Capillary leak caused by local histamine release

Fig 1.3 Skin prick test.

Patients with a history of anaphylaxis should be referred to secondary care for assessment. There is little to be gained by skin testing these patients before referral, and it is among this group that any adverse reactions may occur.

If pressed on the possibility of adverse events, it is worth noting that, in a large North American epidemiological study, there were fewer problems from skin prick testing than from venepuncture.

1.15 Can skin tests be done in a primary care setting?

Skin prick testing was widely performed in general practice before the restrictions imposed on the use of injection immunotherapy in 1986, and it was only the withdrawal of allergen manufacturers from the market place that led to skin testing dying out in primary care. Training for primary care staff in the testing and interpretation of skin prick tests is available from the National Asthma and Respiratory Training Centre in Warwick. (See list of useful contacts in appendix.)

1.16 What diagnostic equipment is appropriate for a general practice?

A modest range of diagnostic allergen extracts, including tree and grass pollens, house dust mite, cat, dog and horse dander, will cover most eventualities. Practices wishing to develop their interest in allergy may wish to extend this list to cover nuts, moulds, cow's milk and egg allergens. Suitable extracts are currently available from the suppliers detailed in the Appendix.

Skin test lancets should be used in preference to hypodermic needles. Hypodermic needles are designed to penetrate the skin rather than create a standard sized breach in the skin for introducing the allergen extract. Moreover, there is a risk of needlestick injury because of the hollow needle. The lancets can be metal or plastic, and generally have a 1-mm angled point. One lancet should be used for each drop to avoid cross-contamination.

1.17 What is the difference between atopy, sensitization and allergy?

Atopy is the genetic trait that confers an increased risk of sensitization. Currently, atopy is assessed by looking for evidence of allergic sensitization. Allergic sensitization means that the subject has detectable IgE directed against relevant allergens, but there may not be any associated disease. Allergy is reserved to describe people who have clinical symptoms as the result of allergic sensitization.

1.18 What types of allergy testing are available?

The idea behind allergy testing is to find out whether a particular substance is capable of causing the symptoms experienced by the patient. Direct challenges of the nose and airways are technically possible, but only one agent can be tested at a time, and several weeks have to be allowed for the target organ to return to baseline before the next agent can be tested. Skin and blood tests serve as surrogates and allow multiple agents to be tested at once. However, the demonstration of allergen-specific antibody in blood does not necessarily mean that the patient will get symptoms upon allergen inhalation. Similarly, skin reactivity does not correlate completely with reactivity of the nose or airways. Thus skin and blood tests require careful interpretation. Direct challenges are the gold standard, but they can only be justified in special contexts such as occupational asthma, where there is no alternative. Oral food challenges can also be performed, but it can be difficult to define an end point, and if the patient's clinical problem is suspected anaphylaxis, there is a significant danger of provoking a full-blown attack.

1.19 Which tests are most appropriate for which patients?

For most immediate-type, antibody-driven allergies, skin testing is the simplest and most effective test. A large number of different extracts can be tested at once, and results will be available within 15 min. Skin tests may be performed on the arms or on the back (generally the arms are preferred in UK allergy clinics). Some patients have very sensitive skin or are unable to stop taking antihistamines, in which case skin testing will be impossible. Blood tests for allergen-specific IgE provide a valid alternative, but cost considerations usually limit the number of allergens that can be tested. Blood tests are also useful in patients with extreme sensitivity and for assessing sensitivity to allergens for which no suitable skin test extracts are available. Patients with eczema and delayed-onset reactions should be assessed by patch tests, which detect cell-mediated contact sensitivity. Patch tests are generally performed on the back, as the test substances have to be applied for 48 h.

1.20 What are the advantages and disadvantages of the different diagnostic tests?

Skin tests are cheap and quick to perform. The results are clear to the patient and relatives, so it is easy to say 'look what cat dander does to your arm; imagine what it does inside you!' The basis of the test is that the skin serves as a surrogate organ. Some patients have very sensitive skin, especially in urticaria, and will react just to scratching the skin or to the diluent used to prepare the extract. A negative control is always included to make sure that the positive reactions are genuine. Other patients are unable to stop their antihistamines, in which case the positive results will not be visible. A histamine solution is used as a positive control to ensure that reactions would be seen if histamine was released. Hence the positive control validates the negative responses and the negative control validates the positive responses.

1.21   What technical factors can affect skin tests?

Weal size varies depending on where the skin test is performed. For example, the skin of the upper arm is looser than that over the wrist area, so the same skin test solution will induce a smaller weal if applied near the wrist than if used near the elbow. Skin test responses vary slightly over the day, and there is a small but definite effect of the menstrual cycle on the size of the weal. These differences are not critical for diagnostic use, but could confuse the outcome of research studies if the timing of tests is not standardized. Antihistamines will reduce or block the weal response.

MANAGEMENT

1.22   What are the management principles for allergic disease?

■ Identification of trigger factors.

■ Avoidance where possible.

■ Drug treatment to deal with residual symptoms, but using the minimum that will achieve maximum/full remission and minimizing the impact of allergic disease on school attendance and work.

As far as possible, patients should be empowered to manage their own care and take back control of their lives.

1.23   When does an allergy problem require referral for specialist attention?

This depends on the expertise of the person seeing the patient. Simple allergic problems can, and should, be handled in the community or in primary care. Specialist back-up may be needed if the patient or their advisor is unsure what to do, or if the patient fails to respond to standard therapy. Specialists are best used to see patients who do not fit the standard guidelines for diagnosis and therapy, or in whom there are possible serious clinical or medicolegal issues (e.g. allergic reactions during anaesthesia, occupational asthma, etc.). Specialist advice should also be sought before starting interventions that may have a major impact on patients' quality of life.

1.24   Is it possible to desensitize people?

Yes, but not every patient with allergic disease is suitable (*Table 1.2*).

TABLE 1.2 Indications and contraindications for immunotherapy

Indications	Contraindications
Treatment of choice	Age <6 years
Wasp and bee venom hypersensitivity	Age >50 years (relative
Valid option	contraindication)
Allergic rhinoconjunctivitis due to grass or	Coronary heart disease
tree pollen	Autoimmune disease
Allergic rhinoconjunctivitis due to cat or	Hyperthyroidism
house dust mite	Beta-blockers
Valid in Europe and US, but not	Current wheeze
recommended in UK	
Allergic asthma	
Not recommended anywhere	
Atopic eczema	
Food allergy	
Drug allergy	
Occupational allergy	

Desensitization aims to reduce the symptoms of allergy by building up the body's tolerance to the allergen responsible for the patient's symptoms. This can be achieved by giving repeated amounts of the allergen, starting with a minute dose and building up at weekly intervals to a maintenance dose, which is then continued every 4–6 weeks for up to 3 years. Once the course of injections is complete, symptoms should remain suppressed for several years, if not permanently. This approach has been widely used for hay fever and other seasonal allergies in the past and, although it is not widely available in the UK for asthma and rhinitis, it remains the treatment of choice for anaphylaxis caused by wasp or bee stings.

1.25 How does desensitization work?

It is not known exactly how it works, but it is known that immunotherapy alters the way in which the patient's immune system reacts to subsequent exposure to the allergen. At one time it was thought that immunotherapy worked by inducing protective antibodies that would intercept pollen proteins and prevent them from reaching the mast cell and triggering histamine release. IgG antibodies are produced during desensitization but, as the mast cells are close to the surface of the mucous membranes and the protective antibodies are much deeper, the antibodies cannot intercept allergenic proteins. Moreover, patients who have received immunotherapy still show immediate skin test responses to allergens. However, after immunotherapy, they do not show any delayed (late-phase) reactions, and it seems that their tendency to develop symptoms has become uncoupled from their sensitivity. In other words, they still have sensitizing antibodies that can trigger a skin test response, but they do not show any delayed reactions and they have substantially reduced clinical symptoms. This process of disconnecting antibodies from symptoms is probably regulated by T cells.

1.26 What advantages might desensitization have over drug therapy?

Desensitization can offer relief where conventional and optimal drug therapy has failed. Whilst the treatment is intensive and may be protracted over several years, it does have lasting effects. Not only can desensitization effectively cure a patient but it may also prevent progression of the allergic condition. For example, there is evidence that treating allergic rhinitis with immunotherapy can halt progression to asthma.

1.27 Is hyposensitization the same as desensitization?

The terms are used interchangeably. Strictly speaking, hyposensitization means reducing sensitivity while desensitization means removing it altogether.

1.28 What are the potential risks and side-effects of desensitization?
(See *Box 1.2*)

 Most patients will have local inflammation at the site of their injections, especially as the doses increase towards the maintenance dose. Some will get large local reactions which develop over several hours and may take 24–48 h to resolve. Rarely, patients may have systemic reactions after injections. These may be mild (nasal congestion, rhinitis) or more serious (urticaria, angioedema, bronchospasm and hypotension). Quite often, patients may have mild and rather non-specific systemic symptoms, such as mild headaches and muscle aches, in the 24 h after injections.

BOX 1.2 Adverse reactions to immunotherapy

- Local reactions in about 7% of patients
- Systemic reactions in about 0.3% of patients
- Most reactions occur at the start of the course or when maximum dose is being achieved
- >75% of reactions occur within 20 min of injection

1.29 Is there any serious danger in desensitizing allergic patients?

Since you are injecting patients with substances to which they are allergic, there is a risk of triggering an allergic reaction. In the past, some patients have died after immunotherapy injections, but fortunately this is very rare and there have been no such fatalities in the UK since 1986. The risk of adverse events can be minimized by following the proper dose schedule, and by avoiding injections when patients are ill with intercurrent infections. Patients with asthma are at greater risk of adverse events than non-asthmatic patients, especially if their asthma is active or poorly controlled at the time of injections. Almost all the documented fatalities after immunotherapy have occurred in patients with asthma, who were being treated for their asthma. Careful attention to checking the dose and assessment of the patient will substantially reduce the risk of adverse events, while prompt treatment will minimize the risk to the patient of any adverse events that do occur.

1.30 What are the differences between diagnostic and therapeutic allergen extracts (and does it really matter)?

Both preparations are made from the same source material. Diagnostic extracts need to contain all the biologically relevant materials. They are then prepared in a concentrated form, in a diluent that contains preservatives, as the extract will be used repeatedly over many months. In contrast, extracts for therapy may not need to contain all the components of the extract to be effective. Therapeutic extracts need to be sterile but they will be used soon after reconstitution, so there is less need for preservative. However, therapeutic solutions are often dilute and so the diluent needs to contain some extra protein (e.g. human serum albumin), otherwise the proteins in the extract will precipitate on the walls of the vial.

1.31 What is a depot preparation and how does this differ from an aqueous extract?

Immunotherapy extracts come in a variety of different forms. Simple extracts made up in water-based buffers are called aqueous extracts. In depot preparations, the allergenic material is adsorbed onto a carrier (usually aluminium sulphate), which allows the protein to be released slowly after injection. As well as reducing the rate of delivery, hence minimizing the risk of side-effects, the aluminium vehicle alters the presentation of the antigens to the immune system. This may affect the cytokine pattern of the subsequent immune response.

1.32 How are extracts standardized and what do all the figures mean?

The potency of allergen extracts can be assessed in the laboratory in terms of their relative composition of proteins and their ability to bind to pooled sera from allergic patients. Alternatively, they can be biologically standardized by testing on a panel of patients who are known to be sensitive to the allergen in question.

Biological standardization allows comparisons to be made between extracts in terms of their ability to elicit a weal response. Ideally, any given patient should show the same sized weal when tested with different batches of the same extract or with extracts from different manufacturers. Moreover, a 10-mm weal to a grass pollen extract should indicate the same degree of clinical sensitivity as a 10-mm weal to cat dander.

In Europe, extracts are standardized relative to histamine by comparing the concentration of allergen that elicits a weal response equivalent to a 10 mg/ml solution of histamine, in a panel of allergic patients. In the US, extracts are standardized in terms of their ability to induce erythema (the flare component of the allergic response). The units are thus comparable but not equivalent. Some manufacturers use their own systems of units; these are usually proportionally related to the biologically defined units recommended by the regulatory authorities.

1.33 For what conditions is desensitization appropriate?

Desensitization is the treatment of choice for anaphylaxis to wasp and bee venom. Desensitization has a place in the management of allergic rhinitis, especially when this is refractory to standard drug treatment. In the UK, desensitization is not recommended when the primary problem is asthma, although in many parts of Europe and North America, asthma remains a valid indication. There is no evidence that desensitization helps in atopic eczema or urticaria. Extracts suitable for desensitizing patients with peanut and latex allergy are currently being developed, but their clinical usefulness has not yet been defined.

PROGNOSIS

1.34 Do allergic children become allergic adults?

Allergic sensitization tends to persist, but symptoms may resolve. Allergy to egg and cow's milk is very common in early childhood, and this commonly disappears by school age. Allergy to peanuts is more persistent, but about 20% of children with peanut allergy will lose it by the time they reach 18 years. The earlier that airborne allergy and asthma appear, the more likely they are to persist into adolescence and adulthood. However, a significant proportion of children with allergic asthma will go into remission and may only have symptoms if they develop respiratory infections. Hay fever commonly starts in late adolescence and persists into adulthood, but may gradually fade as patients approach middle age. Conversely, a significant number of adults with asthma develop their condition without ever having had any definable problems in childhood.

1.35   Does exposure to pollutants worsen allergic conditions?

Many people believe that air pollution is responsible for their symptoms. While there is little evidence that air pollution can cause asthma, it is clear that ozone and particulate pollution can make asthma worse in those who already have the condition. The mechanisms underlying this are complex. Ozone stimulates nerve endings in the lungs, causing difficulty in filling the lungs. This is clinically more important in those with asthma. Ozone also causes inflammation in the airways, and imposes an oxidative stress on the airways lining, which is already subject to excessive oxidative stress in asthma.

Small changes in particulate pollution adversely affect lung function and are associated with increased rates of exacerbation of asthma. However, the inflammatory effects of particles on the airways are more marked in normal healthy subjects than in asthmatic volunteers, suggesting that the mechanisms of sensitivity are more complex than researchers originally thought.

1.36   How likely is a person to develop further allergies if they already have one?

In most people, the risk of allergic sensitization is a general risk, not just confined to a single agent. This means that people who become allergic to something carry the general risk of sensitization, and if they are exposed to other potent allergens in the home or workplace, they will be at increased risk of sensitization. Separately, there are suggestions that having allergic inflammation in your airway will alter the local environment and make it more favourable for the development of allergic-type responses. Sensitizing antibodies can trap allergenic proteins and direct them towards the immune system even when there is insufficient protein to trigger the immune system in a non-allergic individual. Treatment studies suggest that if an allergic condition is treated effectively, this may reduce the chance of becoming sensitized to new allergens. This has been shown in several studies of immunotherapy and has been claimed with drug therapy, albeit on less convincing data.

1.37   Can an allergy that develops in adult life go away?

Yes, it may. Whilst the tendency to develop allergies is permanent, the likelihood of developing new allergies decreases with age, and existing allergies may become less troublesome.

THE FUTURE

1.38   What treatment advances can we expect in the next 10 years?

We now understand a great deal about the inflammatory mechanisms involved in allergic diseases (*Fig. 1.4*). Using this knowledge, several new treatments have been developed that are currently undergoing trials. Most of these are targeted therapies, directed against specific parts of the allergic inflammatory response. Some of these affect several different steps in the allergic process, and are likely to be more effective than those that are very specific to a single step.

Modern genetic technology has allowed us to identify the important components of allergenic proteins, and vaccines have been prepared that contain only the main allergenic elements. These need to be tested for safety and effectiveness, but should make desensitization more predictable. Alternative routes of administration are also being tested, including drops and tablets for oral desensitization.

1.39   How can allergy services be improved?

Perhaps, more importantly, we should expect and demand a better system of healthcare delivery for people with allergic disease. Better use of

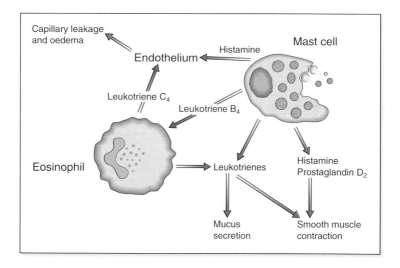

▲

Fig. 1.4 Cells and mediators involved in the acute allergic response.

information technology and more appropriate provision of services in primary and secondary care should allow more people with allergic conditions to receive accurate and effective information about their condition, and hence enable them to make informed decisions about therapy.

1.40 Should I be developing allergy services in my practice?

The primary care sector is in a state of flux at the moment, owing to renegotiation of doctors' contracts and parallel discussions about the future shape of the healthcare system. Whatever shape the new system takes, we can be sure that there will continue to be a large number of patients with allergic conditions who will want to know more about their condition, the substance to which they are reacting, and what they can do to improve matters. Ideally, this advice should be easily accessible to the patient and, with better IT provision, it should be possible to provide targeted information and recommended care pathways for individual patients and their advisors in the healthcare system. Anyone who is advising on allergen avoidance or other targeted intervention ought really to be offering a diagnostic service to guide their decision-making. Many nurses specializing in asthma have already received training in skin testing and allergy advice, but some practices are reluctant to deploy them to fulfil this task as there are other calls on their time and no direct reimbursement. Skin testing is useful and relatively cheap, but may not be an appropriate option for a practice that only tests a few patients each year. Easy access to, and sensible use of, immunological blood tests may be a better option for low-volume users.

1.41 My patient has asked about the 'hygiene hypothesis'. What are the implications of this theory in the prevention and management of allergy?

The hygiene hypothesis brings together a number of different strands that link infection and the risk of developing allergic disease. There are several different versions of the hypothesis, and it must be stressed that this is still a theory, and not something upon which firm advice can be based. The main strands of the hypothesis are:

(1) Allergy has increased in parallel with a reduction in exposure to parasites and waterborne infections.
(2) Some infections and vaccinations may protect against the development of allergy.
(3) Some environmental bacteria present in soil may protect against allergy — the modern emphasis on clean food, refrigerators, etc. may have reduced our exposure to these harmless helpful bacteria.

(4) Food technology and changes in diet have affected our gut bacteria and this makes our children vulnerable to developing allergies.

(5) Bringing up children on farms may be protective against allergies, but only if the children are raised in close proximity to animals (e.g. spending time in the cow byre before the age of 1 year).

However, and in contrast to some press reports, the hygiene hypothesis is not about using too many household cleaners in the kitchen, washing hands, or normal childhood vaccinations.

As of today, there are no specific actions that anyone should take in response to the hygiene hypothesis. Clinical trials are assessing whether artificial changes in the gut bacteria may affect the risk of developing allergies, but it is too early to make any definitive recommendation. Meanwhile, normal standards of cleanliness are recommended. Children should be encouraged to play outside, to eat a balanced diet and to develop normal standards of personal hygiene.

PATIENT QUESTIONS

1.42 Is allergy inherited?

The predisposition to allergies (atopy) is inherited rather than the allergy itself.

The inheritance pattern is complex, and appears to involve several genes, so not all children of atopic parents will inherit the same degree of genetic risk. Allergies occur because of a mixture of inherited and environmental factors. Atopic people seem to react to whatever allergens are in their environment. For example, on the north-east coast of the US, people are allergic to house dust mites; in poorer housing in the south-east, cockroaches are the main allergen, while in the dry air of the Arizona desert, dog dander and the mould *Alternaria* are the main culprits.

1.43 What determines whether an atopic person develops an allergy?

This depends on the timing of exposure, other immunological challenges, adjuvant factors and various co-factors.

- ■ Timing — the earlier in life the exposure takes place the more likely a child is to develop an allergy. Swedish studies have shown that babies born during the birch pollen season are more often allergic to birch than babies born at other times of the year.
- ■ Other immunological challenges — the more colds a child has in early life the less likely they are to develop allergic disorders. (See section on hygiene hypothesis.)
- ■ Adjuvant factors — such factors as air pollution and cigarette smoking enhance an individual's risk of developing allergy. For example, babies born to mothers who smoke are twice as likely to develop asthma at some stage in their life.
- ■ Co-factors — in some people an established allergy can be exacerbated by co-factors such as exercise, cold air, fever, aspirin or certain foods.

1.44 Are allergies very specific?

True allergies are highly specific and involve the recognition by the immune system of highly specific components of the target allergen(s). Some allergic individuals will recognize multiple elements of the target, or multiple targets, but they do this either by making multiple antibodies which each recognize different elements; alternatively, there may be common targets on multiple molecules. The ability to recognize such targets is partly determined by inheritance and partly by exposure.

1.45 What is cross-reactivity?

Some patients who are allergic to one allergen may experience symptoms on exposure to apparently unrelated substances. These reactions can be explained by antibodies that recognize similar structures on the two allergens. The structures on any protein recognized by antibodies are called epitopes.

1.46 Is contact with pets advisable for atopic people?

Generally it is OK to be in contact with pets to which you are not sensitized, but if you buy a pet or work with animals, then atopic people are likely to become sensitized. Accordingly, it is unwise for atopic individuals to go out and buy furred pets. Animal allergens are potent and can be carried on clothing or remain in carpets and furnishings for several months.

Patients who are allergic or who come from allergic families should be encouraged to consider pets which do not shed allergen, e.g. fish and reptiles, or a pet that is confined to a cage and does not spread allergen around the house. Pets such as hamsters, guinea pigs, etc. should never be kept in bedrooms as this dramatically increases the amount of allergen exposure and hence the risk of becoming sensitized.

1.47 What is total allergy syndrome?

Total allergy syndrome and multiple chemical sensitivity are terms used to describe a condition in which the patient appears to experience reactions to a wide range of substances. The patient describes diffuse symptoms, including fatigue, breathing difficulties, loss of concentration and memory, depression and nausea. A wide range of chemicals, fumes and synthetic materials is often implicated by the patient, but no objective tests can confirm this sensitivity. Some sufferers find relief from avoidance of all fumes and chemicals, but at the expense of retreating from normal everyday activities. On conventional criteria, many of these patients exhibit features of agoraphobia and other neurotic illness. Whatever the true cause, the symptoms are very disabling and can prove intractable, both to conventional and unconventional therapies. Despite its name it is thought not to be allergic in origin, and patients do not demonstrate the classic immune responses seen in other allergic diseases.

1.48 Can allergy be responsible for non-specific symptoms such as tiredness and mood changes?

It is fashionable to blame allergy for many different illnesses and problems. Patients with hay fever and asthma may report tiredness and irritability, especially during the height of the pollen season or when taking sedating antihistamines, but allergy is rarely, if ever, responsible for isolated tiredness or mood changes in the absence of any definable allergic condition.

1.49 Can dogs be allergic to humans?

Yes. Dogs and cats can develop a form of atopic dermatitis. This is more likely to be allergic in origin in dogs. The most common type of allergy seen in dogs and cats is to fleas, resulting in flea allergy dermatitis. The allergic reaction is to the flea saliva and typically affects the area around the base of the tail towards the middle of the back. Dogs can also react to human dander, which makes up a high proportion of household dust.

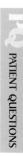

Asthma

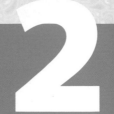

INTRODUCTION

2.1   What is asthma?

Asthma is a clinical condition in which there is transient narrowing of the airways, causing increased resistance to the flow of air into and out of the lungs. Episodes of asthma can be triggered by a variety of factors, some of which affect all patients, others of which are specific to certain individuals (*Fig. 2.1*). Unlike some other respiratory conditions which show fixed narrowing and obstruction of the airways, in asthma the obstruction will resolve either on its own or with drugs that open up the airways (bronchodilators). The degree of improvement with drugs may be complete or partial, leading to the concept of fully reversible or partially reversible airways obstruction.

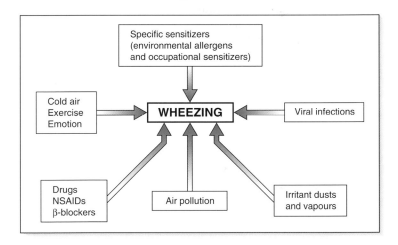

Fig 2.1 Triggers of asthma symptoms.

2.2   Is all asthma the same?

Several distinct clinical patterns are recognized. These are sometimes called clinical phenotypes. Examples include the following:

- Exercise-induced asthma
- Aspirin-induced asthma
- Nocturnal asthma
- Acute severe asthma

■ Brittle asthma
■ Occupational asthma.

Current research is focusing on whether the same mechanisms operate in all these different patterns, and it seems that there are some characteristic differences between them. These differences are important in understanding what causes asthma, for knowing how best to evaluate new drugs, and also for advising on the best type of treatment for each patient with asthma.

2.3   Why is it sometimes called bronchial asthma?

The original Greek term 'asthma' referred to acute episodes of breathlessness. These can be caused by heart diseases, especially left heart failure and mitral valve disease, as well as by obstructive lung disorders. Early physicians distinguished between asthma caused by heart disease, which they called cardiac asthma, and asthma because of airways disease, which they called bronchial asthma, the bronchi being the main tubes carrying air into the lung. The term cardiac asthma is now obsolete, but bronchial asthma lives on!

EPIDEMIOLOGY

2.4   Is asthma becoming more common?

Yes. A threefold rise in the number of children with asthma occurred between 1960 and 1990. Contacts with the GP for asthma have risen fivefold for children aged 5–14 years over this period, while the increase for children aged 0–4 years has gone up by 10 times. Hospital admissions for asthma for these age groups have gone up by 10- and 20-fold, respectively. This means that, as well as there being more people with asthma, something is happening at the health service level which is exaggerating the true rise in asthma. Both the true increase in the number of children with asthma and the use of medical services by asthmatics are now levelling off, but the rates are not yet reducing.

2.5   Why is asthma becoming more common?

When the rise in asthma was first noticed, many medical people thought this might be an artifact caused by changes in diagnostic fashion. In the 1950s and early 1960s, children with asthma were often sent away to special schools, so when a child had mild asthma, parents and doctors would often agree that the child did not in fact have asthma, and would label the illness as 'wheezy bronchitis'. Only those with severe asthma were labelled as asthmatic. This meant that people thought of asthma as being a severe disease, and it also meant that patients with mild forms of asthma did not receive anti-asthma medication. Once inhaled corticosteroids were introduced in 1969, people realized that mild to moderate asthma could be improved, so there was a need to diagnose all cases of asthma properly, so that the patients would receive the right medication. This increased the number of people diagnosed and labelled as asthmatic without any real increase in the number of people who really had the disease.

In addition to this change in diagnostic labelling, there has been a clear increase in asthma, allergic rhinitis and eczema since 1960. The best UK data comes from Aberdeen, where the same questionnaire was used in 1964 and 1989. This showed an increase in childhood asthma from 4.1% to 10.2% over the 25 years. Parallel increases in hay fever (from 3.2% to 11.9%) and in eczema (from 5.3% to 12.0%) suggest that something has happened in one generation that affects the risks of developing all forms of allergic disease, not just the risk of becoming asthmatic. While asthma certainly has a genetic component, one cannot blame a rise of this scale on a change in the genetic make-up of the population, so we must look to environmental causes.

Evidence from Germany indicates that people born in West Germany before 1960 have the same risk of allergic disease as their counterparts born in East Germany. From 1960 onwards a gap started to open up and, in those born in West Germany from 1985 to 1989, there were almost three times as many children with allergic diseases as in the equivalent group from East Germany. Since the fall of the Berlin wall, this gap has started to close. This tells us two important things: firstly, there is something about the western affluent lifestyle that plays a part in making more children develop allergies; and secondly, the risk is defined early in life, and does not alter later, even if the society becomes more and more affluent (*see Question 11.3*).

Several major environmental changes have happened since 1960. Chief among these are changes in housing design (e.g. double glazing, better insulation, central heating, fitted carpets, all of which favour the growth of house dust mite), increased pollution from increased traffic, changes in food technology, and reductions in the dirtiness of the environment in which our children grow up. There are plausible arguments in favour of each of these, but it is likely that there are several factors involved and probably different factors apply to different extents in different people.

2.6   Is pollution responsible for asthma?

Old fashioned forms of pollution caused by burning coal for electricity and domestic heating have declined considerably since 1960. There has been a small but definite increase in other forms of pollution in recent years. Ozone can trigger asthma attacks in people who already have the condition, but is not thought to be capable of causing asthma in otherwise healthy people. Particulate pollution has been implicated in cardiovascular and respiratory problems, and diesel exhaust particles may influence the risk of becoming sensitized to pollen allergens. Overall, there is some evidence that air pollution makes asthma worse, but no real evidence that pollution is responsible for causing asthma.

2.7 What is the role of allergy in the development and maintenance of asthma?

Sensitization to airborne allergens is an important risk factor for the development of childhood asthma. However, it is less clear whether allergy is responsible for maintaining asthma. On the one hand, it is possible to reduce the irritability of the airways by extreme allergen avoidance measures; however, conventional allergen avoidance measures have very little impact on asthma symptoms.

2.8 Is all asthma allergic?

No. Up to 80% of children with asthma show signs of allergies, but allergies are much less frequent in adults with asthma. Even in children, where allergic sensitization is a clear risk factor, it is less clear whether the allergies are responsible for the maintenance of the condition (*see Question 2.7*).

2.9 Does wheezing in infancy lead on to asthma?

Wheezing is very common in the first 2 years of life. Most often this occurs with viral respiratory infections and it seems that those with smaller lungs are more likely to wheeze than those with larger lungs. However, up to the age of 18 months, there is no relationship between infantile wheezing and the subsequent development of allergic asthma. Of course, some of those who wheeze in the first 18 months of life will go on to develop asthma, but statistically these children are no more likely to go on to develop asthma than children who have never wheezed.

Among those children who are atopic, the risk that wheezing will persist is much increased compared to non-allergic children.

DIAGNOSIS

2.10 How is asthma diagnosed?

Asthma is primarily a clinical diagnosis, which is supported by measurements of airflow obstruction. The clinical history will give a pretty clear picture, but thought should be given to excluding other conditions that cause episodic breathlessness and cough, including cystic fibrosis, antibody deficiency, chronic bronchitis, heart failure, anaemia, etc. There may be wheezing in the chest during acute attacks, but the chest may sound completely normal between episodes.

2.11   Which investigations are useful in diagnosing asthma?

Serial measurements of peak flow rate are simple to perform and will show up characteristic morning dips in most patients with asthma. Some patients may only show peak flow variability during episodes, so a normal peak flow chart does not completely exclude asthma. Simple spirometry may show a reduced forced expiratory volume in one second (FEV_1) and a relatively normal forced vital capacity (FVC). Patients with some degree of airflow obstruction may show reversibility when given a dose of bronchodilator (e.g. two puffs of a salbutamol inhaler). This is more reliably shown on spirometry than by peak flow rate, and a 15% improvement is taken as the minimum that can be regarded as confirming asthma. In cases of doubt, bronchial challenge tests may be useful (*see Question 2.12*).

2.12   Are bronchial challenge tests useful?

There are two types of bronchial challenge (bronchoprovocation) tests: allergen challenges with something to which the patient is sensitized and non-specific airway challenges using histamine or methacholine, to which everyone responds, but to which asthmatics are more sensitive.

Allergen challenge causes a brisk narrowing of the airway (*Fig. 2.2*). There may simply be an acute reaction or there may be a biphasic or dual response with immediate and late-phase bronchospasm (*Fig. 2.3*). Allergen challenges are useful for research into the mechanisms of asthma or in testing new drugs, but they are too cumbersome for routine clinical use, except in occupational asthma where no alternatives exist. Airways irritability is a hallmark of asthma, so in clinical practice a non-specific airway challenge can be useful to rule out asthma, but a positive test does not prove asthma. In research work, non-specific challenges can be used to grade the degree of airway irritability.

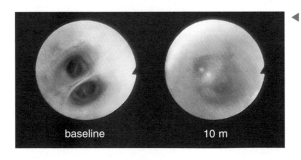

Fig 2.2 Effect of allergen challenge on asthmatic airway. Bronchoscopic view of right middle lobe bronchus before and 10 minutes after allergen challenge.

baseline   10 m

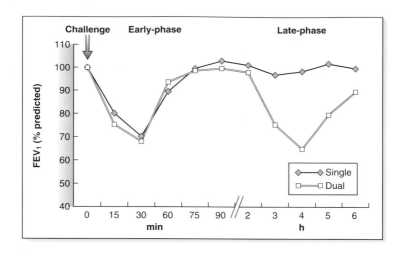

▲

Fig 2.3 Response to allergen inhalation.

2.13 Is skin testing useful in the diagnosis of asthma?

All patients with asthma should be assessed for possible risk factors and trigger factors, including the role of allergies in triggering their symptoms. Skin testing is a valuable means of assessing whether patients are sensitized to house dust mite, domestic animals, etc. Nobody should spend money on mite avoidance measures or get rid of their pets without first undergoing skin tests to confirm whether these allergens are in fact relevant in their particular case. Interpretation of skin tests requires some skill and care: skin tests should always be interpreted in the context of the clinical history, and the measures proposed should be proportionate both to the degree of symptoms and to the strength of the skin reactions (*see Question 2.20*).

MANAGEMENT

2.14 What are the principles of managing asthma?

See *Box 2.1*.

2.15 What are the virtues of a stepwise approach to asthma?

A wide variety of drugs are used to treat asthma (*Box 2.2*). A stepwise approach to asthma enables patients and doctors to arrive at the appropriate level of treatment for asthma, as well as structuring decisions on treatment changes. Following an initial assessment of severity, patients

BOX 2.1 Management of asthma

- Accurate diagnosis
- Empowerment of patients and their families to care for the condition
- Minimizing symptoms and allowing patients to lead as normal a life as possible
- Minimizing absence from school and work through appropriate avoidance measures and appropriate use of therapy
- Minimizing the risk of side-effects

BOX 2.2 Drugs used to treat asthma

- Corticosteroids
- β-adrenergic bronchodilators
    Short-acting, e.g. salbutamol, terbutaline
    Long-acting, e.g. salmeterol, formoterol
- Leukotriene receptor antagonists
- Theophyllines
- Anticholinergics (ipratropium, oxitropium, etc.)
- Immunomodulators
    Methotrexate, cyclosporin A, etc.

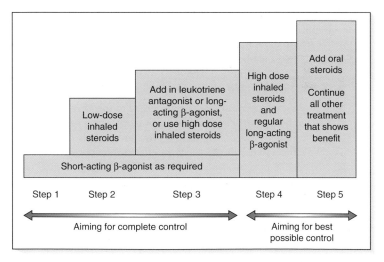

Fig 2.4 Stepwise management of asthma.

are started on the step that seems most sensible (*Fig. 2.4*). Their progress is reviewed periodically, and their anti-asthma medication is increased in a structured manner until good control is achieved. Assessment of control is generally judged by a combination of symptoms and peak flow rate charts. Once the patient is stable, they may need occasional step-ups to cover exacerbations, but they should revert to their usual maintenance dose on recovery from the exacerbation. Monitoring should be continued and, if symptoms are well controlled for 3 months or more, then a step-down in therapy should be considered. Long-term anti-inflammatory medication should only be withdrawn in patients who have been stable and effectively symptom-free for at least 6 months. Most patients who require regular anti-inflammatory therapy will need to continue this indefinitely. The stepwise approach thus helps to set the initial dose for anti-asthma therapy, guides the patient to their optimal maintenance dose, and encourages the use of the minimum amount of medication that is required to control the disease.

2.16 How can we empower patients?

See *Box 2.3*.

2.17 Are there any special features of asthma at school?

Asthma is common at school age, and in most children it should be quite easy to control. Conflicts can arise around sport and physical exercise, and some children will use their asthma as an escape mechanism. Good relationships between the child, their parents and teachers will help to avoid or minimize the risks of manipulative behaviour.

Access to inhalers during school should be fairly free, although some regulation is reasonable. Careful and appropriate staff training is required

---

BOX 2.3 How can we empower patients?

- Providing information that is appropriate to their needs
- Giving them control of their medication, including rescue medication for exacerbations, and providing the advice necessary to enable them to use the medications effectively
- Not making patients dependent on medical and paramedical services
- Encouraging independence, but responding rapidly to calls for help
- Praising the patient for calling for help when appropriate
- Reinforcing advice about what to do if their condition deteriorates
- Avoiding statements that encourage dependency (e.g. saying that they might have died if they had not called for help, etc.)
- Accepting the role of facilitator rather than paternalistic carer and source of knowledge — something that is quite hard for most healthcare professionals!

to allow teachers to distinguish between genuine need and inappropriate or disruptive use of inhalers. If managed properly, asthma should not lead to loss of school attendance. If significant amounts of school loss are occurring, the patient needs formal medical assessment by a specialist paediatrician to see whether the asthma could be better managed, or whether other factors are responsible for absence from school.

2.18 Persistent asthma in a non-compliant teenager: what really works?

Talking to teenagers about what might happen to them when they get old is unlikely to have much impact. Most teenagers think that everyone over 20 is irretrievably ancient, and the idea that they should worry about what they will be like when they are 30 or 40 is totally irrelevant. However, teenagers are heavily influenced by their peers, and one of the reasons they are reluctant to take medication is that they do not want to appear different (or weaker) than their peers. Different strategies work to a greater or lesser degree in different teenagers, but some options include:

- Avoiding overmedicalization. Who wants to play the sick role when they should be out there chasing boys/girls, playing music and having fun?
- Giving the teenager responsibility for their condition.
- Most teenagers with asthma were children with asthma, and their parents have often taken responsibility for managing the condition. Parents can find it difficult to let go and allow the child to manage their asthma, especially if they don't seem to be doing it as well as Mum or Dad would.
- Divorce the paediatrician: show the teenager that they are now the boss and that they report to their own doctor/nurse, not to the paediatrician chosen by their parents.
- Demonstrating that by managing their asthma better, they will be able to do more, and to keep up with their peers.
- Telling the teenager that there is a good chance their asthma will decrease or even go away if they look after it properly, but treating them as adults and being honest if they ask questions.
- Engaging the teenager in the choice of medication will often lead to them choosing a device that they like for its engineering or its colour and, provided it works and they want to use it, who cares which one they use!
- Having an adult discussion about smoking and asthma.
- Asking them about what they want to do when they grow up and whether they have concerns about how asthma might interfere with their ambitions.

2.19 How can one control exercise-induced wheeze?

Many children and adults with asthma experience wheezing on exertion. People with asthma often avoid exercise, and can become very unfit, so not all breathlessness on exertion in asthmatics is really exercise-induced wheeze! Exercise-induced wheeze is more likely in cold and dry conditions. Swimming is the form of exercise least likely to trigger this wheeze. Exercise-induced wheeze can be completely prevented by taking a leukotriene receptor antagonist half an hour before exercise. Using salbutamol 10 min before exercise also has some benefit.

2.20 Is allergen avoidance helpful in the management of asthma?

Up to a point! Extreme levels of allergen avoidance can reduce mite exposure and improve symptoms. For example, sleeping in a hospital ward each night or spending several months at altitude will lead to a reduction in bronchial irritability and asthma symptoms in mite-allergic patients. However, it is difficult to separate off the effect of a long holiday at altitude on general happiness and wellbeing from the effect of the reduction in mite exposure that is achieved by going on holiday at altitude!

Allergy is a risk factor for the development of childhood asthma, so most asthmatic children will have positive allergy skin tests. However, so do 30% of the healthy non-asthmatic population. Thus, it is not true to say that the presence of positive skin tests automatically means that allergy is responsible for the patient's symptoms. In general, the stronger the degree of sensitization shown by the skin test, the more likely it is that the allergy may be contributing to current symptoms. If someone is very allergic to house dust mite, domestic animals, etc., it makes sense to reduce exposure in the hope that this will either improve current symptoms or reduce the risk of longer term immunological damage. Conversely, nobody should undertake allergen avoidance measures without first having their allergic status assessed.

2.21 How can house dust mite be avoided?

House dust mites are present in high numbers in bedding and sofas, where their need for heat and humidity are best met. Closely woven fabrics are available which will allow air and moisture to cross, but will prevent the mites and their faecal particles from crossing the fabric barrier. Covering mattresses, duvets and pillows with close-fitting covers made from this type of fabric will substantially reduce the local concentrations of house dust mite antigens. Removing other dust reservoirs such as carpets, soft toys, cluttered surfaces and heavy fabric curtains will reduce exposure. Frequent vacuum cleaning will help, but care should be taken to avoid resuspending dust. Most modern vacuum cleaners have integral filters which prevent recirculation of dust. In terms of dust resuspension, there is little to choose between modern vacuum cleaners, but they are all significantly superior to pre-1990 models in this respect. Vacuuming is not a substitute for removing carpets; if carpets are essential, it is preferable to have loose rugs, which can be taken outside and cleaned, or fabric mats that can be washed, rather than fitted carpets.

2.22   What is aspirin-induced asthma?

Aspirin sensitivity is not an allergy, but a reaction to the way that the drug works. Aspirin's main function is to block an enzyme called cyclo-oxygenase (COX), which helps to convert a fatty acid called arachidonic acid into inflammatory chemicals called prostaglandins. Prostaglandins are responsible for many different processes in inflammation, including the stimulation of pain fibres, so by blocking their production aspirin reduces inflammation and discomfort. There are several forms of COX and the critical enzyme for pain is COX-2. Aspirin is quite a crude drug, and it also blocks another COX enzyme called COX-1. When COX-1 is blocked, inflammatory cells start to convert arachidonic acid into another type of inflammatory chemical called leukotrienes. Leukotrienes cause asthma, rhinitis and urticaria, so if patients who are sensitive to leukotrienes take aspirin, they will trigger attacks of their asthma. The same thing happens if the patient takes any other form of drug which inhibits COX-1. This includes almost all the other non-steroidal anti-inflammatory drugs (NSAIDs) because they work in the same way as aspirin, and so they will also trigger attacks in people with aspirin-sensitive asthma. There are over 20 different such NSAIDs, but the commonest ones to cause trouble are ibuprofen (Nurofen) and diclofenac (Voltarol), because these are the most widely prescribed NSAIDs. Many foods also contain aspirin-like compounds, called salicylates, that can also trigger symptoms in some aspirin-sensitive patients.

2.23   How is aspirin-induced asthma managed?

Obviously the patient should avoid aspirin and related drugs, although it is in fact possible to desensitize aspirin-sensitive patients temporarily if for some reason it is essential to use aspirin on a regular basis. The desensitization lasts as long as the patient continues to take the same dose of aspirin, but tolerance can be breached if the dose is increased or stopped. Until recently, management consisted of avoidance of NSAIDs and prescription of a low salicylate diet, but the recent introduction of leukotriene antagonists has provided a very precise tool that specifically targets the responsible mechanism. While taking a leukotriene antagonist, the patient should be able to eat a completely normal diet, but it is still best to avoid COX-1 inhibitors.

2.24 What painkillers can aspirin-sensitive patients take?

 There are now selective COX-2 inhibitors (rofecoxib and celecoxib) which can be safely used to treat arthritis and inflammation in patients who are sensitive to leukotrienes. Paracetamol is usually safe but can cause trouble in some patients who are very sensitive to aspirin. Codeine-type painkillers should be safe, although some patients are sensitive to codeine, quite independently of aspirin sensitivity.

2.25 Can asthma be caused by infections?

Viral respiratory infections are a common trigger of attacks in children who already have asthma and to a lesser degree in adults with the condition. In fact, viral infections in early life seem to protect against the development of asthma, possibly by deviating the immune system away from the allergic-type response and towards a more protective pattern of response.

One special form of asthma is associated with fungal colonization of the airways. This condition is called allergic bronchopulmonary aspergillosis (ABPA) and is caused by a complex reaction against the mould *Aspergillus fumigatus*. Unlike standard asthma, patients with ABPA often have patches of consolidation on their chest X-ray, and may go on to develop permanent damage to the airways and a form of bronchiectasis. ABPA usually responds well to steroids, but these may have to be given systemically to be fully effective.

The role of bacterial infections in asthma is controversial and the subject of current research.

2.26 When should I be concerned about occupational asthma?

In clinical practice there are two quite distinct contexts:

1. The possibility of occupational asthma should always be considered in people who develop asthma for the first time in adulthood, regardless of their occupational history. About 10–15% of new onset adult asthma has an occupational component.

2. People who become breathless while working in an industry known to be prone to occupational asthma will often come to their doctor asking if their problem is occupational asthma. Before diagnosing occupational asthma in this group of patients, an accurate exposure history must be obtained, and other forms of heart or lung disease excluded. Most of these industries are taking proper precautions to limit exposure, but sometimes working practices are faulty. In patients who smoke, it may be very difficult to work out what proportion of the patient's breathlessness is due to asthma and what proportion is due to smoking.

2.27   Which occupational groups are most at risk?

Work-related asthma comes in several forms: all patients with asthma will experience symptoms when exposed to dusty workplaces, especially if there are also solvents, endotoxins, etc. This is not regarded as occupational asthma, but is compensatable if the employer has not taken appropriate precautions to reduce the dustiness of the workplace, and to minimize the personal exposure of workers. Classical occupational asthma is defined as asthma caused by sensitization to something encountered in the workplace. The commonest single cause is isocyanates (used in two-pack spray paints, and plastics manufacture). Warehouse workers and others handling organic dusts are often affected, the commonest group being bakers (who may be allergic to flour and the amylase enzyme used to improve flour). About 10% of laboratory animal handlers become allergic to proteins in the urine of rodents. Other industrial processes with high rates of asthma are platinum refining, electronics (solder fluxes and acid anhydrides), and welding.

2.28   If I am concerned about occupational factors how should I proceed?

Ideally, arrange for the patient to make peak flow recordings for 2 weeks while at work and for a similar period while away from work. Measurements (best of three blows) should be made every 2 h while awake. All values should be recorded by the patient and then plotted out by medical staff, not the patient. The sensitivity of such recordings is much greater if done while the patient is still exposed in the workplace. In many cases, the patients will have been removed from exposure pending a decision on whether they do or do not have occupational asthma, and the employer may be reluctant to allow them back to work to make peak flow recordings.

A detailed occupational history is needed, including details of all dusts and chemicals encountered in the workplace. Detailed assessment of exposure is beyond medical expertise, but can be performed by an industrial hygienist if needed for medicolegal reporting. Before taking someone out of the workplace for good, they should be referred for assessment by an expert in occupational asthma, as the diagnosis can be difficult and the economic impact of removing someone's livelihood when they do not in fact have occupational asthma is enormous. In cases of doubt, or when a new agent is suspected, formal bronchoprovocation challenges should be performed (by an appropriately trained expert).

2.29   Will patients with occupational asthma improve if removed from the workplace?

Roughly one-third will lose their asthma completely, one-third will show clear improvement, and one-third will not improve at all. Failure to improve does not mean the diagnosis of occupational asthma is wrong. Rather it seems that the asthma process is started off by the occupational exposure, but then the inflammatory process becomes independent and continues without needing the inciting agent to be present.

Factors associated with better prognosis include a shorter period between development of symptoms and time of diagnosis, less severe asthma at the time of diagnosis, and rapid removal from exposure. Patients who continue to be exposed for more than 1 year after developing occupational asthma are very unlikely to make a full recovery.

2.30 How quickly following removal from the workplace will patients stabilize?

Lung function will stabilize within 12–18 months of removal; bronchial irritability takes a little longer to settle. Thus, assessment at 2 years after removal from exposure will give a pretty accurate picture of the residual level of symptoms and airflow obstruction.

2.31 Does prompt treatment with steroids affect the outcome of occupational asthma?

It is generally believed that early use of steroids will help speed recovery but there is little hard evidence to support this belief. For the time being, the symptoms of occupational asthma should be managed exactly as per standard treatment guidelines, the only major philosophical difference being the insistence on eliminating or reducing allergen exposure.

2.32 What career advice should I be offering to a 14-year-old with allergic asthma?

Some careers are barred to asthmatics. These include the armed services and police force, who are reluctant to train people with a history of asthma, as they are more likely to drop out of the physical training programmes. Baking and paint-spraying specifically exclude asthmatics, and anyone with allergies to animals should think twice about training as a vet, as a veterinary assistant or as a laboratory worker.

2.33 Is there a role for desensitization in asthmatic patients?

Desensitization works in some patients with asthma, but it carries significantly higher risks of adverse reactions in patients with asthma (as opposed to patients with rhinitis but no asthma), so the selection of patients likely to benefit is a critical issue.

Before considering desensitization one has to be convinced: (1) that allergic sensitization is an important factor in the continuing level of symptoms; and (2) that all reasonable measures have been taken to reduce exposure. If the patient remains symptomatic, then the critical question is whether the residual symptoms are driven by one or more inhaled allergens. If there was no tangible benefit from reducing house dust mite exposure, then one should be sceptical that house dust is relevant in that particular patient. However, where there is a clear link between exposure and symptoms (e.g. casual exposure to cats) and no further avoidance measures can be taken, then there may be a good case for desensitization. The case for desensitization may be enhanced if the patient also has allergic rhinitis which has not responded to standard therapy. The more severe the asthma, the less effective desensitization will be, so the ideal candidate is someone who has a high degree of sensitization as shown by skin tests, mildish asthma and more severe rhinitis.

2.34   Is complementary medicine useful in asthma?

Understandably, many people with asthma want to find some explanation for why they have developed asthma, and some way of controlling their condition. This can make patients vulnerable to suggestions from a wide range of informed and uninformed opinion. Alternative allergists may use unconventional techniques to diagnose trigger factors for asthma or may prescribe unconventional treatments for asthma. The value of these approaches varies from patient to patient: crudely, those who believe in this approach are likely to gain more benefit in the short term than those who are sceptical.

2.35   Are complementary medicine diagnostic techniques useful in asthma?

A wide range of techniques is being used to try and determine trigger factors for asthma. Usually the patient will be told that they are allergic to the substances in question. This use of the term allergic is the lay usage (as in 'I'm allergic to Monday mornings') rather than the medical and scientific sense of there being immune recognition of a foreign substance that causes an allergic reaction. As discussed elsewhere (see Question 12.3) we have to assume that the alternative practitioner believes in the validity of what they are doing, otherwise they would be guilty of fraud. However, there is no hard evidence that any of the electrical, physical, reflex or analytical techniques have any value in diagnosing trigger factors for asthma.

2.36   Is there any value in complementary medicine treatment for asthma?

Many people with asthma are understandably frustrated that conventional medicine cannot offer them a cure, and so they seek out additional advice and therapy. Some of the benefits of complementary medicine are because the therapist appears to have more time to spend with the patient than the standard NHS service allows. Other benefits probably relate to the uncritical stance taken by the alternative therapist. Most of us are more convinced by someone who says they know exactly what is needed, as opposed to some self-critical doctor who says that they do not know what works best, so they will have to guess or else conduct a clinical trial. Most patients play both sides of the street, but some unscrupulous alternative therapists try to persuade patients that they must stop all conventional therapy if the alternative therapies are to have any chance of working. At best this is nonsense, and at worst it can lead to disastrous destabilization of asthma through inappropriate withdrawal of effective and necessary medication.

2.37 Can diet be a contributor to asthma?

Allergy to eggs and cow's milk can cause a variety of allergic symptoms in children, and clearly should be avoided by those with obvious multisystem allergies. Some foods contain aspirin-like substances called salicylates that can trigger asthma attacks in patients who have aspirin-sensitive asthma. However, the amount of salicylate in food is quite small. Blackcurrants are listed as containing high amounts of salicylate but you have to eat 2 kg of blackcurrants to consume the equivalent of one junior aspirin! The best way to test for this condition is by a trial of a leukotriene receptor antagonist (montelukast or zafirlukast) rather than by starting a diet. It is certainly true that people who are experiencing anaphylactic shock to peanuts, etc. will wheeze as part of their anaphylactic episode, but there is no real evidence that food allergy causes isolated asthma in adults. Careful analysis of large series of cases shows that patients who have asthma, but do not have any symptoms in or around the mouth, will not react to foods when formally challenged in the laboratory.

2.38 Is it better to take anti-asthma drugs in the morning or evening?

Asthma is typically at its worst in the early hours of the morning, when the body's cortisol levels are lowest. Most anti-asthma drugs are given twice daily, on rising and on retiring. Long-acting bronchodilators are best used at night, when they will continue to act across the worst period. Anti-leukotriene drugs also seem to work best when given at night.

PROGNOSIS

2.39 Does childhood asthma really disappear?

Yes.

Most children with asthma will lose it by the time they are 18-years-old, but in some cases it will come back. Of 100 children with asthma at age 7 years, 35 will go into complete remission, five will have asthma continuously through to the age of 33, and the remaining 60 will have intermittent asthma, usually but not always, triggered by episodes of viral respiratory infection.

2.40 Does the early use of inhaled steroids make a difference to the long-term outcome of asthma?

Although this has been claimed, the data are really inconclusive. The most widely quoted study compared two groups of children, one of which was started on inhaled steroids immediately while the other group was left for 2 years and only received steroids if their doctor thought it was necessary. When those in the second group were started on inhaled steroids after 2 years, they did not respond as well as the group who had been given steroids immediately upon diagnosis. However, many of those who started off in the second group dropped out of the study, so the group that was given steroids after 2 years was quite different to the group that started off in the study. The correct interpretation of the work is that it was inconclusive as the two groups were not matched, but it has been widely quoted as evidence by those who believe in giving inhaled steroids at the first sign of asthma.

2.41 What is meant by airways remodelling?

In asthma, the airways are altered by the inflammatory reactions that take place and, as a result, the airways behave differently to those of non-asthmatic people. The term 'airways remodelling' has been used to describe this, but tends to mean different things to different people. At its broadest, it refers to the changes that occur in asthma which lead to altered physiological responses to non-immunological triggers such as exercise, smoke, perfumes, etc. Other people restrict the term to describe scarring processes that are seen in the airways of people with long-term asthma. The alterations described as airways remodelling include:

- Changes to the physical structure of the airway (*Fig. 2.5*; damage to the epithelium, swelling of the lining of the airway, loss of elasticity in the airway wall, collagen deposition in the airway wall).
- Changes to the functioning of structural elements of the airway (enhanced contraction and decreased relaxation of airway smooth muscle cells; increased mucus secretion from glandular cells in the airway lining and wall).
- Changes to the local immune system (increased amounts of cytokines biasing towards an allergic pattern of response; re-routing of foreign

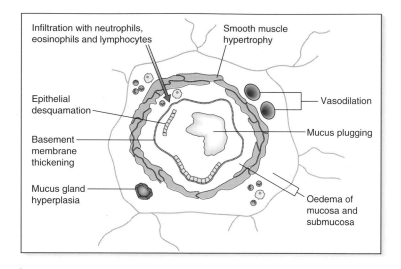

Infiltration with neutrophils,
eosinophils and lymphocytes

Smooth muscle
hypertrophy

Epithelial
desquamation

Vasodilation

Basement
membrane
thickening

Mucus plugging

Mucus gland
hyperplasia

Oedema of
mucosa and
submucosa

▲

Fig 2.5 Inflammatory changes in the airways in chronic asthma.

material to the immune system; deposition of cytokines on matrix proteins and their subsequent release by proteases).

■ Gradual loss of reversibility of airflow obstruction, either by the development of pharmacological tolerance or by the onset of fixed airway obstruction.

2.42 What happens eventually to the airways of people with asthma?

Most people with asthma lead lives of normal duration with minimal disability, although a significant proportion do experience some limitation in their exercise capacity as a result of their asthma. A small proportion go on to develop fixed airway obstruction, although this is largely confined to those who smoke, and it is not entirely clear whether the asthma or the smoking is really responsible for the change in the clinical pattern over time.

2.43 How likely are patients to die from asthma?

Fortunately death from asthma is relatively rare considering the number of people who have the condition, but a small number of patients do die from asthma each year. It is difficult to obtain accurate figures because of overlap with chronic obstructive pulmonary disease, especially in older people, but a best estimate is somewhere between 1200 and 1500 deaths from asthma of people aged between 5 and 40 in the UK each year. The total number of asthma-related deaths has been falling in recent years, despite the increased number of people with the condition, suggesting that current management strategies are reducing the risk of acute asthma proving fatal. Moreover, the risk of fatal asthma is largely confined to patients with more severe forms of the disease, and the bulk of the rise in asthma has been at the mild end of the spectrum. Some risk factors for asthma death can be identified: patients with a history of unstable asthma or previous life-threatening attacks; patients who delay seeking help when their asthma deteriorates; allowing medication to run out or go far beyond expiry date. Once in the emergency medical setting, fatal outcomes from asthma are associated with delays in giving systemic steroids, and with failure to recognize exhaustion and respiratory failure. Appropriate use of ventilatory support will often buy time to allow the patient to start on the road to recovery. In the most severe cases, artificial ventilation will restore normal blood oxygen levels and allow the exhausted respiratory muscles time to recover.

THE FUTURE

2.44 What new concepts in the management of asthma are likely to emerge over the next 5–10 years?

Clinically, the trend is to recognize that there are, in fact, several different types of asthma, each of which has different risk factors and may require different management strategies. This means that treatment and management packages should be tailored to individuals rather than taking a 'one size fits all' approach. As well as the clinical diversity, there may also be genetic differences in patients' ability to respond to different anti-asthma drugs. This might allow treatments to be chosen on the basis of suitability to the individual's genetic make-up (pharmacogenetics).

If suitable targets emerge from the current series of research programmes, it may be possible eventually to identify molecular targets that are involved in the persistence of asthma, and hence offer the possibility of curing the disorder rather than simply containing it as is currently the case.

2.45 Will monoclonal antibodies like anti-IgE be useful?

Monoclonal antibodies have been developed that are directed against the sensitizing IgE antibodies. Unlike the older forms of anti-IgE antibody, which could trigger allergic-type reactions, these new antibodies 'see' IgE that is free in the bloodstream, but cannot recognize IgE that is bound to effector cells (mast cells and basophils). These new anti-IgE antibodies can be used as a research tool to find out which bits of asthma (or other allergic conditions) are really driven by IgE. To date, anti-IgE looks as if it may be

helpful in some patients with more severe asthma, but it is unlikely to be
cost-effective in milder forms of asthma unless it can be shown to abolish
the disease and, as yet, there is no evidence of this.

2.46   **Which other molecules are being considered as possible targets
for treating asthma?**

Over the past 15 years, a wealth of knowledge has emerged about the cells
and molecules involved in asthma. However, ask four clinical scientists
which molecule is the most important one and you will probably get at least
four, and probably more, different answers. The major targets under
consideration are:

■ Cytokines involved in the development of allergy (IL-4, IL-13).

■ Molecules involved in the recruitment and activation of inflammatory
leukocytes (adhesion molecules, chemokines, including eotaxin, IL-4,
IL-5).

■ Proteases released from inflammatory cells (tryptase, etc.).

■ Molecules that regulate the growth and repair of epithelial cells.

■ Molecules that regulate the function of airway smooth muscle cells.

2 / Asthma **47**

 PATIENT QUESTIONS

2.47 For how long should I breast feed to protect my child from developing asthma?

There is no evidence that continuing breast feeding beyond 6 months of age offers any protection against the development of allergies.

Children of atopic parents are at increased risk of developing allergies and asthma. The single most useful thing that an atopic mother can do is to avoid smoking during pregnancy or the first year of her baby's life. Early weaning onto solid food should be avoided and, if breast milk is insufficient, it is probably better to use hydrolysed soy feeds rather than cow's milk-based formula.

2.48 What about exercise?

Exercise is a good thing, and all asthmatics should try to achieve and maintain a good level of physical fitness. Swimming is the form of exercise least likely to trigger wheezing. If exercise-induced wheeze is a recurrent problem, a leukotriene receptor antagonist should be taken half an hour before exercise.

2.49 What is the role of food additives in asthma?

Certain foods and food additives have chemical effects on asthma. These include:

- Sulphites: these are widely used to prevent discoloration of white wine, coleslaw, etc.
- Salicylates: aspirin-like compounds present in many foods in varying amounts.
- Histamine: present in red and white wine, salami, cheese, tuna, salmon, etc.
- E numbers are not harmful in their own right, but should be seen as a practical way of describing food additives without requiring a dictionary and labels a yard long.

2.50 How useful are ionizers and dehumidifiers?

At present there is no evidence that ionizers are helpful and, if they contribute to the humidity in the house, they may actually be harmful by improving the living conditions of the resident house dust mites. Dehumidification is helpful if the relative humidity can be reduced to below 40%, as this inhibits the growth of dust mites. However, this is almost impossible to achieve with UK housing stock, as the houses are not sealed and so the humidity levels rapidly return to normal owing to recirculation of air (and damp) from outside. In cold climates, such as Canada and Scandinavia, where houses are triple-glazed and relatively 'airtight', many houses have complete climate control systems which can regulate temperature and humidity in different parts of the house. In this context, dehumidification has been enormously helpful in reducing the tendency for

PATIENT QUESTIONS

mould growth in winter, and may also have helped to reduce mite growth, although there has been a parallel move towards hardwood flooring which also helps to reduce mite exposure.

2.51 Should we get rid of our pet if our child is asthmatic?

If someone is allergic to a domestic pet, then ideally the pet should go, as its continued presence will hamper recovery and may cause increased damage. It is common for patients to report that their pet does not affect them but other people's pets do. In part this is wishful thinking, but it also reflects the fact that in homes that contain pets, the pet allergens will be very widespread throughout the house, on clothing, carpets and soft furnishings. This means that the level of pet exposure in the home will be pretty constant whether the pet is present in the room or not. On entering another dwelling, the patient may detect the contrast between the levels of pet allergens that they are used to, and the higher levels in the house being visited.

2.52 What extent of contact with pets is acceptable?

People with allergic parents or siblings are more at risk of becoming sensitized than those without any family history of allergy. Anyone who is allergic to one pet is likely to become allergic to other animals if they are sufficiently exposed. Sensitization is more likely with increasing exposure, and particularly if there are high levels of allergenic material in the bedroom. It follows that all animals should be kept out of the bedroom, even if the affected person is not there. If an allergic person is contemplating purchase of a pet, consider fish, or perhaps adopting an animal at a nearby zoo, as parting with one's pets is much harder than not buying them in the first place.

2.53 Are some dogs more allergenic than others?

From an immunological point of view, all dogs are identical, and there is no evidence of any breed-specific antigens. However, there may be some difference in the amount of dog allergen that is shed by different breeds, either as the result of different hair length or differential secretion of sweat and sebum on the skin surface. Male cats secrete more cat allergen than females, and it is possible that similar gender differences also exist in dogs.

2.54 Which jobs can I do if I am asthmatic?

People with asthma can do most types of work, but should avoid workplaces that are very dusty or have heavy exposure to fumes and solvents. Asthmatics are excluded from certain occupations by health and safety legislation (e.g. paint spraying, baking and platinum refining) because of the high risk of developing further sensitization. The police and armed services generally decline applications from people with current asthma, and in some cases from people with a history of asthma, because they are more likely to fail to complete the required physical fitness programmes. Also, if accepted, they are more likely to be invalided out. Access to civilian work with these services is not affected.

2.55 Why are there such great country to country variations in the management of asthma?

The clinical management of any condition is a complex product of the availability of medications in that country, the health beliefs of patients, their relatives and their doctors, as well as political and cultural factors which vary from place to place and time to time. In the UK we are comfortable with devolving responsibility for asthma care to patients, and within the primary care team to nurses. In other healthcare systems, doctors are paid according to how many patients they see with each condition, so there are incentives to see patients more often, and to retain control of the patient and their illness. This may not be a conscious decision by the doctor, and is often dressed up as the doctor saying that it is better for the patient to be reviewed frequently by a doctor. Drug availability and reimbursement schemes affect prescribing decisions; e.g. inhaled steroids were not available in the USA until 1987, so patients with bad asthma were managed on oral steroids, while those with moderate disease were given theophyllines much more often than in Europe and Canada.

Hay fever

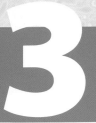

INTRODUCTION

3.1 What is the natural history of hay fever?

Hay fever typically starts in late childhood or young adulthood, with a peak in the teenage years. A minority of sufferers develop their symptoms for the first time after the age of 30 years, but some care is needed before labelling rhinoconjunctivitis as hay fever when it appears for the first time in middle age. People who move from one country to another may experience a honeymoon period, usually 2–3 years, when they do not get symptoms from their hay fever. This happens because they are not exposed to the pollens that have previously caused their hay fever, and it takes 1–2 seasons for them to become sensitized to pollens in the new area. As time goes on, many sufferers find that their hay fever symptoms become less troublesome. This reflects a gradual reduction in all forms of immunity from the age of 18 years onwards. While this causes some reduction in people's ability to fight off infections as they age, it also allows IgE levels to fall gradually and hence reduce clinical sensitivity to pollens. Separately, the sensitivity of the end organs (nose and eyes) to inflammatory mediators may also reduce over time. This is clearly seen in the skin, where responses to histamine decline with age, and similar effects are thought to occur in the eyes, nose and lungs. In some patients there is loss of seasonality, either because of the development of sensitivity to perennial allergens (*see Question 3.5*) or because fixed nasal obstruction develops.

3.2 Are there any serious sequelae?

Not really. The main long-term effects are social, e.g. public examinations generally take place during the peak hay fever season and this may adversely affect the performance of students with hay fever, both directly because of the circulating inflammatory mediators and indirectly as a consequence of the side-effects of medication. Other possible risks include adverse effects from immunotherapy (*see Question 3.23*) and an increased risk of developing asthma; however, it is not clear whether treating hay fever helps to reduce this risk.

DIAGNOSIS

3.3 What are the salient features of hay fever?

See *Box 3.1*.

3.4 When should investigations be considered?

Most patients who have the usual symptoms during the grass pollen season will not need any form of investigation. Patients with perennial symptoms

---

BOX 3.1 Features of hay fever

Seasonal conjunctivitis and/or rhinitis occurring typically during the season of grass pollination

Itchy, sticky eyes

Bags under the eyes

Sneezing; watery rhinorrhoea

Nasal blockage

Postnasal drip and itch at the back of the throat

Seasonal cough and wheeze

Symptoms are usually worse on sunny days or if driving with the car window open. Symptoms may also be worse in the evening (see peak pollen levels)

---

should not be labelled as having hay fever, but should be investigated for perennial allergies or fixed nasal obstruction. The diagnosis should also be reconsidered in patients with atypical eye symptoms or epistaxis.

Any patient who is being considered for immunotherapy should undergo specialist assessment prior to commencing treatment.

3.5   Why do some patients start off with seasonal hay fever and then get year round symptoms?

This can happen for two distinct reasons, and both reasons can apply in some cases. Firstly, patients who are initially sensitive only to grass pollen may develop additional sensitivities. If these new sensitivities are against allergens which are present all year round, then their clinical picture may shift from well defined seasonal allergic rhinitis to a more perennial picture. The commonest agents to do this in the UK are house dust mite and cat dander. Alternatively, the patient may develop structural changes in the nose, which leave them with permanent obstruction. The commonest cause of this is the development of nasal polyps, which are very common in patients with allergic rhinitis, whatever the initial trigger. Other patients may develop intrinsic rhinitis (*see Question 4.2*), either spontaneously or as the result of chronic inflammation caused by repeated exposure to allergic insults over many years.

MANAGEMENT

3.6   What is the best strategy for managing hay fever?

As with any allergy, the general principle is to avoid triggers where possible, and to use the minimum amount of effective medication to control residual symptoms.

Patients with mild occasional symptoms should use antihistamines as required. Most of these can be bought over the counter, although this is relatively expensive compared to the costs of prescription charges. For preference, use long-acting, non-sedating antihistamines (*see Question 3.11*). If the symptoms are more persistent, a topical nasal corticosteroid spray (NCS) should be used. Aqueous preparations provide better coverage of the nasal mucosa than the older aerosols. There is little to choose between the different aqueous preparations, but some patients find one type preferable to another, so it is worth trying a different brand if the first choice fails to achieve the required effect. NCS sprays work best when used regularly, ideally twice a day on rising and retiring. If there are breakthrough symptoms, additional medication should be given (i.e. as well as the NCS). Itch, sneezing and conjunctivitis respond to antihistamines; rhinorrhoea responds to the anticholinergic Rinatec (ipratropium spray) and nasal blockage may improve with short-term use of decongestants (*Fig. 3.1*). If blockage does not respond to NCS or decongestants, a diagnosis of fixed nasal obstruction should be considered and a rhinological opinion obtained.

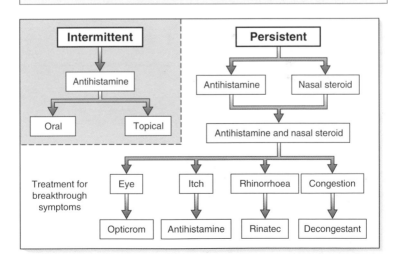

Fig 3.1 Stepwise management of hay fever.

3.7 Is it possible to avoid exposure to grass pollen?

Up to a point. Peak pollen levels occur after 10 am on days when the sun is shining. Typically, pollen is released in the first 2 hours of sunshine after 10 am (i.e. it will be delayed if it is dull early in the day). Pollen rises in the air to altitudes of up to 20 000 feet and then descends as the air cools. In the country, this leads to a rise in ground level pollen concentrations around 6–9 pm, but in cities the air stays warmer for longer and the peak ground level pollen concentration may not occur until between 9 pm and midnight. In other words, in the country you will have problems sitting outside country pubs in the evening, but in town you will have problems coming home from the pub or if you sleep with the windows open after a sunny day.

Planning outdoor activities around these timings will help reduce the impact of hay fever. Other tactics include wearing sunglasses while outside or driving, driving with the windows shut (ideally with air conditioning that includes a pollen filter).

3.8 How are pollen counts generated and where does one find accurate calendars and predictions?

Pollen counts are generated by measuring the number of pollen grains (*Fig. 3.2*) in a specified volume of air, using a pollen trap which draws in a known volume of air, and then literally counting how many pollen grains are trapped. For practical purposes all grass pollen grains are treated as

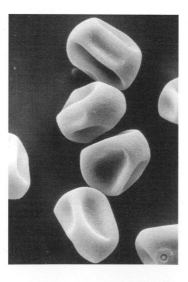

◀ **Fig 3.2** Pollen grains of Timothy grass. © Science Photo Library, reproduced with permission.

similar, but obviously the relevance of the pollen counts will vary according to whether the patient is sensitive to one or more grasses. The precise date of the pollen season is remarkably constant from year to year. There is a distinct South:North gradient, with the onset of the grass pollen season about 2 weeks earlier on the South coast as compared to Scotland. Accurate pollen counts and forecasts may be found at www.pollenuk.co.uk.

3.9 How should one interpret and use pollen counts?

People with hay fever can use the predicted pollen counts to plan their activities. On days when the pollen count is predicted to be high, they may wish to schedule any outdoor activities early in the day or in the early afternoon, avoiding the peak times for pollination.

3.10 What over-the-counter medications are available?

All antihistamines that have been on the market for over 1 year are now licensed for sale over the counter. Newer antihistamines are usually licensed for prescription-only use to start with, but should be allowed over-the-counter status once their initial post-marketing period is safely negotiated. One NCS spray is also available (beclomethasone). In addition, there is a wide range of proprietary alternative remedies for sale in pharmacies. None of these is as effective as the standard therapy and some of them are unlikely to have any true therapeutic effect beyond placebo, but for the patient who prefers milder forms of complementary therapy, these remain an option.

3.11 Which antihistamines are best?

For preference, use long-acting, non-sedating antihistamines such as loratadine, desloratadine, cetirizine, levocetirizine or fexofenadine. Older generation antihistamines such as Piriton (chlorpheniramine) and Atarax (hydroxyzine) are less powerful and have significant sedative effects. In terms of antihistamine potency, desloratadine is about 10 000 times more powerful than chlorpheniramine. This does not mean that it works 10 000 times better than Piriton, but it can sometimes work where the older antihistamines have not proved effective. When tested in driving simulators or psychometric experiments, older antihistamines cause sedation in everyone, but only about 30% of patients are aware of this effect. The effect is seen mainly in terms of temporary lapses of concentration while performing low-skill repetitive tasks, and on instrument monitoring tasks, i.e. tasks similar to long-distance motorway driving or operating machinery. Moreover, the older antihistamines interact with alcohol, so that half a pint of beer may have the same effect on concentration and driving as that normally achieved after 2–3 pints of beer. This increases the risk of accidents, even when the driver is under the breath alcohol test limit. The only advantage is that they are cheap per tablet, but this is offset by the need to use them more often. Some patients prefer short-acting antihistamines (acrivastine) or antihistamine drops, because they feel these start to work quicker, but there is really very little difference in the speed of onset.

3.12 Should we be interested in the non-histamine effects of antihistamines?

Many claims have been made that particular antihistamines have extra anti-allergic effects unrelated to their antihistamine activity. Most of these effects are only seen *in vitro* at concentrations that are not achieved in normal clinical use. While these observations are interesting at the research level, they have no bearing on the choice of one drug over another for routine clinical use.

3.13 Some first generation non-sedating antihistamines had potentially serious side-effects. Have these problems been overcome?

All modern antihistamines were developed from a line of compounds that were pharmacologically dirty. This lineage has given us the psychotropic phenothiazines, local anaesthetics and a number of antihypertensive agents. Earlier drugs often carried taints of their parentage, and so some early antihistamines penetrated the brain and caused sedation, or had effects on the heart. The introduction of terfenadine and astemizole in the early 1980s was a great advance as these were the first antihistamines that did not cause sedation to any clinically apparent degree. Astemizole was very long-acting and tended to cause weight gain, but terfenadine was a great success and became the number one drug worldwide. However, when taken in overdose, terfenadine can affect the heart, causing an unusual cardiac rhythm disturbance called torsade de pointes. It turns out that terfenadine can block a calcium-dependent potassium channel and, if the plasma drug concentration rises above a certain level, this affects the stability of the heart muscle fibres. Unfortunately, terfenadine is a prodrug and is metabolized by a cytochrome p450 enzyme that is vulnerable to inhibition by co-administration of several other drugs, most notably erythromycin and ketoconazole. Several instances of torsade de pointes were reported in patients who had taken normal doses of terfenadine and added in antibiotics or antifungals that they had in their medicine cabinets. The last straw for the regulators came when it emerged that grapefruit juice can also inhibit the cytochrome p450 enzyme.

3.14   If patients can still experience sedation with non-sedating antihistamines how does one manage the patient whose job demands high levels of vigilance?

The US Navy, Federal Aviation Authority and NASA are all happy for pilots to use loratadine or desloratadine, as these have been shown to have no detectable effect on concentration or instrument monitoring tasks. If they are OK on the Space Shuttle they should be OK on the M62 or the M25, or when operating machinery.

3.15   Are systemic steroids useful for severe hay fever?

Yes, in selected cases and situations. Uncomplicated hay fever will respond very well to systemic steroids. So, when someone with bad hay fever is about to get married or about to undertake some important task which requires them to be completely free from symptoms, a short course of oral steroids is a highly effective way of knocking hay fever on the head. Single short courses of oral steroids are almost harmless but obviously if they are given repeatedly over long periods the usual side-effects will apply.

3.16   Is it safe to use depot steroid injections to treat hay fever in the patient who requests them?

There is no doubt that depot steroids work, but there is real concern about their long-term side-effects. Although this may seem like a single injection to cover the season, the biological impact is equivalent to the use of any other form of medium-term systemic steroid. Patients should be encouraged to use topical steroids and modern antihistamines and, if these do not control their symptoms, immunotherapy should definitely be considered.

3.17   What are the side-effects of depot steroids?

Systemic corticosteroids cause problems in two distinct ways: (1) they have direct effects on metabolism and blood pressure because of their difference from endogenous steroids and their use in supraphysiological amounts; and (2) they suppress endogenous production of steroids from the adrenals, thereby reducing the body's ability to respond to stress. The main clinical problems are thinning of the skin and bones (accelerated osteoporosis), impaired glucose tolerance leading to central obesity and diabetes, and reduced resistance to infection.

Depot steroids are no different from oral steroids in their ability to cause these problems, but they are insidious in that the patient and the doctor may think that they have only had 'a single shot for the season'. Most of the side-effects of steroids are directly linked to their ability to influence inflammatory processes, so the more that systemic steroids are used to suppress hay fever, the greater the degree of short- and long-term side-effects. A few side-effects are unrelated to the anti-inflammatory effects of steroids, and a major challenge for the pharmaceutical industry is to produce steroids which are clinically useful without carrying the risk of side-effects.

3.18 Is it better to use nasal drops or nasal sprays?

For most purposes nasal sprays are perfectly adequate and have the advantage that they are easier to store and to administer. Nasal drops are generally reserved for use where the sprays have not been effective, and they offer the advantage of longer dwell time in the nasal cavity and hence better coverage of the nasal mucosa, especially in situations where the nose is congested or blocked.

3.19 When should patients with hay fever be referred for specialist assessment?

In most patients with hay fever the diagnosis is clear, but a specialist opinion should be obtained if there is doubt about the diagnosis, or atypical features.

Referral to a specialist should be considered for anyone who does not achieve satisfactory symptom control with standard therapy (antihistamines and nasal corticosteroid sprays), and also for anyone who experiences intrusive side-effects (e.g. recurrent epistaxis with nasal steroid sprays).

3.20 Are decongestants ever indicated?

Nasal decongestants can be useful in the short term, especially when the nose is so blocked that it is difficult to administer nasal steroid sprays. The principal role of decongestants is as part of a treatment strategy, and they should not be regarded as a solution in their own right. If decongestants are continued beyond about 2 weeks, they gradually become ineffective and the patient may develop rebound congestion, which is attributed to alterations in vascular tone in the nose. Thus it makes sense to start other anti-rhinitis medication with the decongestants, and then withdraw the decongestant once the topical spray is able to penetrate the nose and do its job.

3.21 Why do antihistamines have little effect on nasal blockage?

Nasal congestion is caused by a combination of vascular dilatation, mucosal inflammation and tissue oedema. Some of this is driven by histamine, but several of the cells and mediators involved are driven by other inflammatory mediators and are thus not sensitive to antihistamines. In contrast, local itching and much of the systemic component of rhinitis is histamine-dependent, and hence will respond to antihistamines.

3.22 Is allergen immunotherapy effective and for whom is it appropriate?

Injection immunotherapy consists of a course of injections of pollen extracts, starting at a very low dose and escalating gradually over several weeks, followed by maintenance injections for 2–3 years. This form of therapy was pioneered in London in the late 19th century, but was adopted much more enthusiastically in the US and Europe than in the UK. There is a considerable body of evidence that immunotherapy is effective in patients with hay fever, even in those who are poorly responsive to standard drug therapy. The critical questions are not whether it works, but whether it is safe and cost-effective. Recently, healthcare providers have tended toward the view that hay fever is not economically important and therefore it is not worth spending much money on it. Others feel that hay fever has a significant and largely unrecognized impact on wellbeing, school performance and productivity; moreover, there is new evidence that immunotherapy may reduce the risk of developing new sensitivities and of developing asthma.

3.23 Is allergen immunotherapy safe in hay fever patients?

In general, immunotherapy is safer in those who do not have asthma. A few fatalities have occurred after immunotherapy, and virtually all of these were in patients who had asthma and were being treated for asthma. Consequently, the medical and governmental guidance is that immunotherapy should be considered only in patients with allergic rhinitis which is poorly responsive to standard therapy and who do not have significant asthma. Other important contraindications are coexistent immunological disease (which may be exacerbated by therapy), neoplastic disease (immunotherapy could affect the way in which the immune system handles cancerous cells), treatment with beta-blockers (these block the effect of the adrenaline that is used to treat adverse reactions), or pregnancy (adverse events with hypotension may prejudice the fetus).

PROGNOSIS

3.24 Does allergen immunotherapy alter the prognosis of hay fever?

Yes, in two different ways.
First, immunotherapy can suppress hay fever, and the benefits may last for many years after the therapy. This contrasts with drug therapy, which works while it is given but has no lasting benefit after discontinuation. More importantly, patients who are monosensitized and receive immunotherapy may avoid becoming sensitized to other allergens.

3.25 Does allergen immunotherapy prevent the onset of other allergic diseases?

It seems so. As discussed above, young patients with monosensitivity show a much lower rate of developing further sensitizations if they are given immunotherapy. The mechanisms are not clear but it is likely that, by using immunotherapy, one may alter the airways mucosal microenvironment away from a pro-allergic milieu toward a milieu which is less favourable to the development of allergic responses to allergens that are encountered.

3.26 Is it safe to use topical nasal steroid sprays for long periods?

Although some patients experience nosebleeds after using steroid nasal sprays, most tolerate these preparations very well.
There is no evidence that nasal steroids will thin the mucous membrane lining of the nose or increase the rate of nasal infections.

THE FUTURE

3.27 How realistic is the possibility of a cure for hay fever within the next decade?

Sadly, there is no immediate prospect of a permanent cure. Plans to develop better forms of immunotherapy have focused mainly on safety rather than efficacy. However, several lines of research are looking at new ways of enhancing the efficacy of specific immunotherapy as well as methods of general immunotherapy that might switch off allergic mechanisms whatever the specific cause.

PATIENT QUESTIONS

3.28 Does air pollution affect hay fever?

Modern air pollutants such as ozone, oxides of nitrogen, and fine particles, certainly affect patients with asthma more than normal healthy subjects. However, there is very little hard evidence relating to hay fever. From a theoretical perspective there are three ways that pollution might affect hay fever. First, pollution might increase the risk of becoming sensitized; second, pollution may increase the risk of sensitization translating into clinical symptoms; and third, pollution may affect the likelihood that hay fever progresses to asthma. There is epidemiological evidence that people who live close to major traffic arteries are at increased risk of becoming sensitized to pollen, and that they have higher than expected rates of hay fever; however, there is no convincing evidence that pollution influences the likelihood of progression to asthma.

3.29 Which pollens occur at which time of year? (*Fig. 3.3*)

The pollen season starts with tree pollens, among which birch, hazel and alder are the earliest to appear, sometimes as early as February in the South of England. Later flowering trees include oak, plane and ash during April. Grass pollination starts in the second week of May along the South coast and spreads North over about 2 weeks. Peak grass pollen levels are found during June and then fall back during July. Weed pollens and moulds are found in

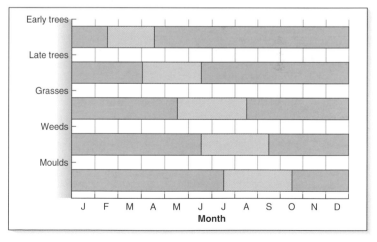

Fig 3.3 Seasonal allergen calendar.

late summer and autumn. Hay fever symptoms may not follow the pollen count exactly, because the amount of pollen required to cause symptoms is greater at the start of the season. This is because the nasal mucosa is primed to respond by the presence of mucosal inflammation. Weed pollens are found throughout the summer, with the same general pattern of pollination earlier in the South and later in the North. Some allergenic plants, such as *Parietaria*, are at the Northern extremes of their botanical range and are only found in the South of England. Pollination seasons are significantly advanced in the Mediterranean and retarded in Scandinavia compared to the UK.

3.30 When should treatment be started for maximal hay fever relief?

Most hay fever treatments work better if they are started before the start of the pollen season. This is partly because the effects of histamine are easier to antagonize if there is antihistamine on board before the histamine is released and partly because, when the nose starts to react, it becomes inflamed. Once the nose is inflamed, it is (a) more difficult both to get topical steroid into the relevant part of the nose, and (b) the nose becomes 'primed' so it will respond to smaller amounts of pollen than were needed initially to cause symptoms.

3.31 How safe are antihistamines in pregnancy and breast feeding mothers?

Following the thalidomide debacle, most companies are reluctant to authorize the use of their drugs in pregnancy. Like most drugs, new antihistamines are not tested formally for use in pregnancy and if you read the package insert it will usually advise against the use of any drug in pregnancy. In so far as the evidence exists, current antihistamines appear to be safe in pregnancy. This is based mainly on the experience gained with hydroxyzine (the parent compound of cetirizine) which was in widespread use from 1968 onwards. However, antihistamines can be concentrated in breast milk and so should not be taken by lactating mothers.

3.32 Can hay fever sufferers get exam dispensations?

There are two distinct ways that hay fever can adversely affect exam performance: hay fever itself can cause a systemic effect through circulating histamine, which makes people feel shabby and febrile; secondly, some antihistamines cause sedation (*see Question 3.11*) which will impair both revision and examination performance. Some concessions are allowed, but these are strictly limited. In principle, it is better to give students optimal therapy and enable them to perform on a level playing field than to allow them to go into exams with a disability.

Perennial rhinitis

4

PQ PATIENT QUESTIONS

INTRODUCTION

4.1 What is meant by perennial rhinitis?

Originally this meant rhinitis which was present all year round and did not change during the pollen season. However, some patients with year-round rhinitis experience substantial seasonal increases in their symptoms, while in some parts of the world the grass pollen season can last for most of the year. As a result, the terminology has recently been revised and people now talk of persistent rhinitis or intermittent rhinitis, without prejudice as to whether there is any season involved. The features of rhinitis are shown in *Table 4.1*.

4.2 How often is perennial rhinitis due to allergy?

Roughly 50% of year-round rhinitis is allergic in origin, usually due to house dust mites or domestic animals.

In patients whose symptoms are truly year-round, with no seasonal exacerbation, about half will have allergic rhinitis while the other half will have a form of non-allergic rhinitis. Some of those with non-allergic rhinitis will have structural problems of the nose and sinuses, and others will have vasomotor rhinitis.

4.3 What are the common allergens involved?

House dust mites are by far the most important allergen in the UK. Cat dander is the next most frequent problem. Small rodents such as hamsters, guinea pigs, rabbits, mice and rats are potent sensitizers, especially if they are kept in children's bedrooms, but numerically these are less of a problem than cats because fewer homes have rodents than have cats.

4.4 Does rhinitis affect the chest?

There is a clear association between rhinitis and asthma. This operates on several levels. Firstly, allergy is a risk factor for both conditions. Secondly,

TABLE 4.1 Features of rhinitis		
Symptom	Seasonal	Perennial
Obstruction	Variable	Predominant
Secretion	Watery, common	Seromucous, postnasal drip
Sneezing	Always	Variable
Loss of smell	Variable	Common
Eye symptoms	Common	Rare
Asthma	Variable	Common
Chronic sinusitis	Occasional	Frequent

rhinitis commonly precedes asthma and it has been suggested that, because having a blocked nose leads to mouth breathing, allergens and other particles may have better access to the lower airways than they would if the patient had a clear nose. Thirdly, the inflammatory process in the nose may influence the behaviour of the airways, both physiologically and immunologically. This may be driven by a combination of neural feedback loops and cytokine growth factors (especially IL-5, inducing systemic eosinophilia and eosinophil activation). Other mechanisms may stimulate airways mucus production, in parallel with the nasal sinus responses. Finally, infected material from the sinuses may drip down into the airway and cause bronchial inflammation. This can be shown in rabbits, but has not been substantiated in humans.

4.5   What are the mechanisms of nasal disease?

The nose is an extremely vascular organ which operates as a heat exchanger and filter. Cold air entering the nose flows past the turbinates, where particles and bacteria are impacted on the mucous membrane. Heat exchange is achieved by drawing the air across vascular beds underneath the mucous membrane. In response to cold, the venous beds become engorged, which limits air flow and increases the availability of warm blood for heat exchange. Instability of vascular tone allows venous engorgement to occur in response to relatively small changes in air temperature or humidity, leading to the clinical picture of vasomotor rhinitis. Infection of the paranasal sinuses causes inflammation and blockage, which in turn cause local sinus pain and prevent drainage of infected mucus. Structural abnormalities of the turbinates and nasal septum allow small changes in the thickness of the nasal mucous membranes to cause more blockage than they would if the bony structures were normally positioned. Allergic reactions cause increased blood flow, mucosal swelling (oedema) and increased mucus production, all of which contribute to nasal blockage and nasal discharge (rhinorrhoea).

4.6   What other nasal problems present in a similar way to perennial rhinitis?

Vasomotor rhinitis is the commonest non-allergic problem to present in this way. Nasal polyps are also common and should be suspected when someone who used to get seasonal rhinitis loses the seasonal pattern of their symptoms.

4.7   What is the role of allergy in sinusitis?

Most sinusitis is caused by infection of the mucus in the paranasal sinuses. This may occur as a primary problem, or may follow blockage of the small holes (ostia) that drain the sinuses into the main nasal cavity. Allergic inflammation is one of the causes of obstruction of the openings of the paranasal sinuses, and hence sinusitis is more common in people with allergic rhinitis than would happen by chance. There is some controversy about whether allergies can be the primary cause of sinusitis and sinus pain. Certain foods affect the bloodflow through the nasal mucosa and hence can make sinusitis worse. However, these foods act directly on the small blood vessels (e.g. biogenic amines (nitrogen-containing compounds found in fermented products: wine, salami, cheese, etc.), sulphites in wine and amines in chocolate).

DIAGNOSIS

4.8 Is it possible to diagnose perennial allergic rhinitis on history alone?

The diagnosis of perennial rhinitis can be made on the history, but diagnostic tests are needed to assess the presence and importance of allergic sensitization.

4.9 Is the patient's diet relevant?

Many patients are concerned that dietary factors may play a role in causing perennial rhinitis. However, there is no evidence that allergy to foods is relevant. Some doctors believe that dairy products can increase mucus production and recommend reducing dietary intake of dairy products for chronic catarrh. If this works, it must presumably be through an effect on mucus glands, or possibly through reduction of biogenic amines in cheese and other fermented milk products, since there is no evidence that antibodies directed against cow's milk play any part in causing or triggering rhinitis.

4.10 Is allergy also involved in the development of nasal polyps and sinusitis?

The combination of nasal polyps, aspirin sensitivity, sinusitis and non-allergic asthma was described by Virchow in the late 19th century (shortly after the discovery of aspirin). These patients are highly sensitive to leukotrienes and, as far as we can tell, the problem is not allergic, even though many of the same mechanisms that are involved in allergy apply. Patients with chronic persistent allergic rhinitis can develop polyps, but this is much less common than in people who are aspirin-sensitive.

4.11 Are skin prick tests useful in perennial rhinitis?

Yes. Skin tests can help to assess the relevance of allergic triggers and can help guide decisions as to whether to undertake allergen avoidance measures. Those who are non-allergic can be saved the cost and trouble of attempting allergen avoidance, while those who are sensitive can be given a more precise opinion on the likelihood of improvement. Specific desensitization is only appropriate in those with proven allergy to relevant allergens.

4.12 Are blood tests for IgE useful in perennial rhinitis?

Measuring allergen-specific IgE can help support a clinical diagnosis of allergic rhinitis. As with skin tests, blood tests will pick up a substantial number of people who make IgE antibodies against house dust mite without developing symptoms, so the blood test results need to be backed up by the clinical history before deciding that specific interventions are indicated. Measurements of total IgE will detect individuals with a general atopic tendency, but this test is much less specific and sensitive than specific IgE measurements: many patients with clinically significant allergic rhinitis have normal total IgE levels, and many healthy people have total IgE levels above normal without disease.

4.13 Is early diagnosis important?

Opinion varies. It has been argued that, if rhinitis is diagnosed early and treated aggressively, this may prevent the onset of other allergies. Some preliminary data in children suggest that those with house dust mite allergy are less likely to become sensitized to other allergens if they receive early treatment with specific immunotherapy.

4.14 Why does intermittent seasonal rhinitis sometimes become persistent?

There are really two distinct scenarios: the patient may start off simply being sensitized to a seasonal allergen (e.g. grass pollen) and then become sensitized to a perennial allergen (house dust mite, cat, etc.). Alternatively, they may start with hay fever but then go on to develop a structural problem which causes perennial symptoms, the commonest of these being the development of nasal polyps.

MANAGEMENT

4.15 How effective is drug therapy in perennial rhinitis?

Antihistamines and topical nasal steroids should give some benefit in perennial allergic rhinitis but unfortunately are often less effective than in hay fever and seasonal rhinitis (see *Fig. 3.1*). In part this reflects the fact that it is not always possible to be sure that the symptoms are truly allergic in origin. However, even in those with allergic sensitization the response may only be partial, and patients often decide to put up with their symptoms rather than take medication every day.

4.16 How effective is specific immunotherapy in perennial rhinitis?

There is no doubt that specific immunotherapy works well in selected patients. For example, spectacular results can be obtained in those who are very allergic to cats. However, efficacy in house dust mite allergy is rather less impressive, perhaps because, in individual patients, it can be difficult to define what proportion of the symptoms is caused by allergy and what proportion is independent.

4.17 Are diets low in salicylates helpful in perennial rhinitis?

Not really. Before the introduction of leukotriene receptor antagonists (LTRA), it was quite common for doctors to recommend salicylate-free diets for several allergic conditions, to find out whether there was an element of aspirin sensitivity. In general, these diets were not very effective, either because the patient was not aspirin-sensitive, or else because dietary salicylates were not responsible for continuing symptoms in patients who were genuinely aspirin-sensitive. Nowadays, any patient who is suspected of being aspirin-sensitive should be tried on an LTRA. If they improve, this suggests that aspirin sensitivity may be an issue, but it is a lot easier (as well as being more effective and probably safer) to keep the patient on an LTRA rather than restrict their diet.

4.18 When should an ENT opinion and surgery be requested?

Facial pain is not a feature of simple allergic rhinitis and should always prompt referral for an ENT opinion. An opinion should also be sought if nasal obstruction fails to respond to topical steroids, or if polyps are suspected. Similarly, chronic purulent or bloodstained nasal discharge also require surgical assessment.

4.19 Management of refractory rhinitis?

Before labelling someone's rhinitis as refractory to therapy, it is important to check the history and compliance with medication, to ensure that the problem has been properly diagnosed, and that appropriate therapy has been advised and attempted. Try using nasal steroids in a head-down posture or a short course of oral steroids (prednisolone 30 mg/day for 5 days). If this fails, consider an ENT opinion and CT scan.

In some cases, simple measures such as switching to an aqueous steroid preparation may allow the topical steroid to coat the mucosa better. Using nasal steroids in a head-down posture will allow the spray to trickle into the upper part of the nose and may make a surprising degree of difference (*Fig. 4.1*). Oral steroids will relieve the situation if the problem is inflammatory, but failure implies that there is a structural problem.

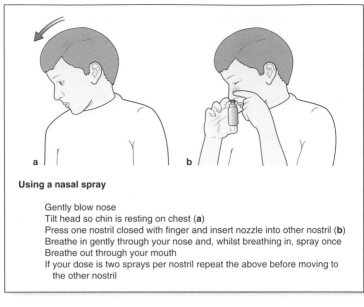

Using a nasal spray

Gently blow nose
Tilt head so chin is resting on chest (**a**)
Press one nostril closed with finger and insert nozzle into other nostril (**b**)
Breathe in gently through your nose and, whilst breathing in, spray once
Breathe out through your mouth
If your dose is two sprays per nostril repeat the above before moving to
the other nostril

▲

Fig 4.1 How to use a nasal spray.

4.20 What works best for nasal congestion?

Topical decongestants are often effective, but should only be used for short periods. Otherwise the nose tends to develop rebound vascular congestion that will not respond to medication. Topical steroids tend to work better against congestion than antihistamines; specific immunotherapy is often effective in those who do not respond to antihistamines and topical nasal steroids.

4.21 Do the same drugs work in allergic and non-allergic perennial rhinitis?

The same drugs are often tried, but antihistamines and topical steroids tend to work better in allergic rhinitis. Anti-leukotriene drugs can be effective in both, and are particularly useful in those patients who are sensitive to aspirin. Ipratropium bromide (Rinatec spray) is useful against watery rhinorrhoea, regardless of allergic status. Allergen avoidance and specific desensitization only work in patients sensitized to the relevant allergen.

PROGNOSIS

4.22 Can perennial rhinitis cause chronic cough?

Many patients with allergic rhinitis experience postnasal drip and associated morning cough. This possibility should be considered in any patient with unexplained chronic cough.

4.23 Does perennial rhinitis lead on to asthma?

Long-term epidemiological studies suggest that a high proportion (perhaps 40%) of people with allergic rhinitis will go on to develop asthmatic symptoms in later life. In many cases, these asthmatic symptoms may be mild and non-troublesome, but in some cases the asthma may come to dominate the clinical picture. Historical evidence suggests that the early use of immunotherapy may prevent or delay the onset of asthma. This has led some to suggest that we should be more aggressive in offering immunotherapy to patients with allergic rhinitis.

THE FUTURE

4.24 Will it be possible to treat mucus hypersecretion more effectively in the future?

Mucus secretion is a common and troublesome feature of rhinitis (and asthma). Agents designed to dissolve or suppress mucus have generally proved disappointing in clinical trials. Current treatments for rhinitis have generally focused on vascular leakage and inflammatory cell recruitment, but there is now a growing interest in the regulation of mucus glands and goblet cells in the mucosa. On past experience, ideas for possible candidate drugs may emerge from this research within 5–8 years, but all will require formal clinical trials and are unlikely to become available for routine prescription until 10–12 years from now.

4.25 Where should we look for a better understanding of the causes of chronic sinusitis?

There is no single satisfactory explanation for chronic sinusitis. Infection is clearly important in a substantial proportion of patients, and may be encouraged by structural abnormalities such as narrow sinus openings that become easily blocked by small degrees of mucosal inflammation. Ciliary dysfunction allows bacteria to persist and cause local damage. This may be because of primary ciliary dysfunction or secondary effects of colonization with bacteria (e.g. *Haemophilus*) that secrete substances that impair ciliary function. Learning how to identify and eliminate such bacteria or how to prevent their effect on the mucosa would clearly be helpful. There is also scope for achieving a better understanding of the relationships between epithelial cell function, mucus formation, mucus clearance and mucosal inflammation.

4.26 Can we expect more effective medical therapy for nasal polyps?

Nasal polyps can be very difficult to manage. Once formed, they are unresponsive to standard drug therapy (e.g. antihistamines and nasal steroids), and will usually require surgical removal. Treatment with nasal steroids has little effect on the recurrence rate after surgery. Since many patients with nasal polyps are sensitive to aspirin and NSAIDs, it has been suggested that leukotrienes may be important in the formation of the polyps. Anecdotal reports suggest that polyps may be less likely to recur if patients receive an LTRA after surgery. Polyp formation may be dependent on growth factors that stimulate the growth of structural cells (fibroblasts), the formation of small blood vessels or the recruitment of inflammatory cells (especially eosinophils).

PQ PATIENT QUESTIONS

4.27 How does one tell whether rhinitis is allergic?

Seasonal rhinitis is usually allergic in origin. Allergic perennial rhinitis is typically made worse by house cleaning (dusting, changing the bed), contact with animals, etc., but these are not reliable and before starting expensive allergen avoidance measures, the diagnosis should be validated by specific diagnostic skin or blood allergy tests.

4.28 How can you help me if my rhinitis is non-allergic?

In the absence of specific triggers, treatment should focus on symptom control. Patients with itch and congestion may improve on antihistamines and/or nasal steroids; patients with watery rhinorrhoea should respond to nasal ipratropium spray; patients with a history of aspirin sensitivity may respond well to leukotriene receptor antagonists.

4.29 Is it safe to take nasal steroids permanently?

Concerns have been expressed that long-term use of nasal steroids may lead to thinning of the nasal mucosa and nasal perforation. These are extremely rare complications, even in those who have used nasal steroids on a regular basis for many years. The risks of systemic absorption have also attracted concern. While it is true that beclomethasone is absorbed and its effects can be detected, there is little evidence that nasal steroids stunt growth or cause long-term damage to bones. Steroids with a high rate of liver metabolism (e.g. fluticasone, mometasone) may be preferable in young people, especially those who are also taking high doses of inhaled steroids.

4.30 Why can't I use a decongestant all the time?

Although decongestants are useful, they can cause permanent damage to the blood vessels of the nose if they are used continuously for long periods. This phenomenon, sometimes called rebound congestion, is thought to be caused by blood vessels adapting to their daily dose of decongestant and becoming tolerant of the drug. This results in the blood vessels opening up again and becoming resistant to the actions of the decongestant.

4.31 Do some nasal steroids cause more nosebleeds than others?

All nasal steroids can cause nosebleeds, and these are reported in about 10% of users. This is a class effect; in other words, the side-effect is common to all steroids. Some patients are more prone than others, and those most affected are likely to have nosebleeds with all the steroid preparations.

4.32 Why do some alcoholic drinks make my nose run or get blocked?

Alcohol is a vasodilator, and some patients are affected by all forms of alcohol. Others only get problems with white wine, with sherry or with brandy. There are two main mechanisms at work. The commonest problem is fermentation products that contain amines. These are found particularly in drinks that were fermented with grape skins present (red wine, sherry, port, brandy etc.). The other problem is from sulphites, which are used to preserve the colour of white wine. Without sulphites, white wine tends to oxidize and turn a pale brownish colour, similar to the flesh of apples that have been cut and exposed to the air. Patients with allergic asthma and rhinitis are often sensitive to sulphites. Most patients with rhinitis seem to tolerate vodka and gin better than they tolerate grape-based alcoholic drinks.

4.33 Why is it that sometimes one side of my nose is blocked and sometimes it is the other side?

Most people (four out of five) have a natural rhythm called the nasal cycle, in which one side of the nose is more clear than the other, then after a few hours the situation reverses. This process is caused by sequential engorgement of blood channels (called venous sinusoids) on one side of the nose, with corresponding shrinkage of the sinusoids in the opposite side. After about 4–12 h the two sides switch. Consequently, most of us do not breathe evenly through our noses, but regularly switch from one side to the other. Of course, some people have structural blockage of one side, either because of trauma (previous broken nose) or because of congenital distorted intranasal anatomy.

Ocular allergy

5

INTRODUCTION

5.1   What allergic eye conditions are there?

There are at least seven distinct clinical entities described. There are the relatively well known conditions of seasonal allergic conjunctivitis, perennial allergic conjunctivitis and acute allergic conjunctivitis. There are then a further three conditions, much rarer and with confusing nomenclature, needing different management and having different prognoses. These are vernal keratoconjunctivitis, atopic keratoconjunctivitis and giant papillary conjunctivitis. Finally, there is contact hypersensitivity or 'allergic contact dermatitis'.

5.2   Do allergic eye problems have common characteristics?

Common symptoms include redness, itching and discharge. Allergic conjunctivitis should be suspected if the eye is itchy. Many patients will report a personal or family history of atopy (asthma, eczema or hay fever).

5.3   How common is allergic conjunctivitis?

Together with blepharitis, allergic conjunctivitis is one of the most common eye conditions managed in general practice. Seasonal allergic conjunctivitis is by far the most prevalent kind of allergic conjunctivitis; however, hay fever sufferers often decide on their own treatment and self-medicate without ever consulting their GP.

5.4   What is the role of airborne allergens in eye disease?

Airborne allergens play a role, but they cannot be held accountable for all ocular allergies. These conditions are usually diagnosed on the basis of clinical appearance, and it is becoming clear that not everyone with the same clinical features will have the same degree of allergic sensitization. Moreover, with an increasing number of people becoming sensitized to airborne allergens (over 30% of adults have a positive skin test to house dust mite), there is a good chance of finding sensitization that is irrelevant to the disease process. This is a casual not causal relationship; in other words, it would not be surprising if 30% of people with painted toenails or NatWest bank accounts are allergic to house dust mite but, as far as we know, there is no causal link. That said, allergic triggers are clearly important in a substantial majority of those with the various eye conditions listed in *Table 5.1*.

5.5   Can non-atopic individuals develop allergic eye problems?

Yes, non-atopic people can develop a cell-mediated contact dermatitis to an allergen. This causes a red, itchy and somewhat scaly reaction of the eyelids and the skin around the eyes. This reaction is usually caused by eye

---

TABLE 5.1 Types and origin of allergic conjunctivitis

Type	Frequent cause
Seasonal allergic (hay fever)	Pollen
Perennial allergic	House dust
Acute allergic	Plants
Vernal catarrh	Pollen
Giant papillary	Contact lens wear
Atopic keratoconjunctivitis	Atopic adult

BOX 5.1 Common causes of periocular contact dermatitis

Topical
      Atropine
      Neomycin
Cosmetics applied to the eyelid
Spectacles
      Metal frames
      Metal hinges and screws
Beauty products
      Perfume
      Hair spray
      Cosmetics applied elsewhere
Chemicals remote from the eye
      Resin adhesives
      Match heads

---

medications, e.g. atropine or neomycin. The reaction will persist as long as the allergen is present.

The metal in spectacle frames can be responsible; the wearers of plastic frames may not be exempt as their metal hinges and screws may also cause problems. Substances without any obvious contact with the eyes (for example, epoxy resins used at work or in leisure activities) may cause problems as they may be inadvertently transferred to the eye by the fingers. Common causes of periocular contact dermatitis are shown in *Box 5.1*.

DIAGNOSIS

5.6 What are the clinical features of allergic conjunctivitis?

Typically both eyes are involved with:

- Intense itchiness of the eyes
- Redness

■ Conjunctival oedema
■ Photophobia

Seasonal allergic conjunctivitis typically occurs in the spring and summer. Perennial allergic conjunctivitis (with symptoms occurring throughout the year) is much less common. The diagnosis is usually straightforward, but one must consider important differentials, such as contact dermatitis, toxic irritant conjunctivitis, foreign body under eyelid and *Chlamydia* infection.

5.7 Can hay fever affect the eyes only?

Occasionally, conjunctivitis is the only sign of hay fever, with no symptoms in the nose at all, so hay fever should not be overlooked as a possible cause of watery red eyes.

5.8 How does one diagnose seasonal allergic conjunctivitis?

Seasonal allergic conjunctivitis (SAC) of hay fever is by far the most common ocular allergy seen. Hay fever often affects the eyes as much as it affects the nose. Indeed, the eye symptoms of hay fever can help to distinguish it from a common cold or from rhinitis caused by other airborne allergens. The eyes are particularly susceptible to pollen as the size and shape of the grains favours their deposition on the conjunctiva. Other important seasonal allergens include tree pollens (typically causing symptoms well before the grass pollen season) and moulds (typically in the autumn). The seasonal pattern is the most important clue to the diagnosis, and most patients with SAC are aware of the allergic basis of their symptoms.

5.9 How does perennial allergic conjunctivitis differ from the seasonal condition?

Perennial allergic conjunctivitis (PAC) is very similar to SAC except that the symptoms and signs are present all year round because the responsible allergen is present throughout the year. In the UK the most common cause is house dust mite, with animal danders (cat, dog, etc.) being the next biggest cause.

Patients will complain of redness, itching and slight mucus discharge throughout the year, but may also describe exacerbations when there is an increase in exposure to the allergic trigger, e.g. changing the bed or spring cleaning (*Box 5.2*).

5.10 What is 'atopic conjunctivitis'?

Strictly speaking it should be the same as allergic conjunctivitis. Just as dermatologists use the term atopic dermatitis to describe a skin disorder that is associated with atopy, so ophthalmologists use the term atopic

---

BOX 5.2 Key features of perennial allergic conjunctivitis

Both eyes involved
Symptoms all year round
Episodic
Household allergen, especially house dust mite
Younger atopic person
Coexistent eczema common

---

conjunctivitis to describe inflamed eyes that look as if they have allergic conjunctivitis. Most, but not all, patients with the clinical condition will also have atopic sensitization. The interesting question is what causes this clinical picture if the patient is not in fact sensitized to airborne allergens!

5.11 Is there value in investigating seasonal or perennial allergic conjunctivitis?

This is rarely indicated. Skin prick testing may confirm the responsible allergen suggested by a detailed allergy history. Eosinophils may be identified on conjunctival smears in half of all patients and IgE levels are usually raised.

In therapeutic trials patients are often given a conjunctival provocation test. The purpose of this test is to determine the minimum allergen dilution that elicits a positive response. Increasing concentrations of allergen are prepared and a drop of each concentration is placed in the eye at 10-min intervals until a clinical reaction is observed. One drop of physiological diluent is administered to the other eye as a control. The clinical reaction is assessed using a standardized scoring system for conjunctival itching, hyperaemia, weeping and nasal blockage.

5.12 Can an acute unilateral red eye have an allergic aetiology?

Curiously, acute allergic conjunctivitis is often unilateral. This very rapid onset follows exposure to a plant such as ragwort. The eye becomes itchy and red, with lid swelling. The extent of the conjunctival swelling can occasionally be so great that the conjunctiva may balloon out between the eyelids. Whilst the rate of onset and the symptoms are alarming to both the patient and their doctor, it resolves very quickly and spontaneously. The patient requires plentiful reassurance but no treatment, although an oral antihistamine may be given.

5.13 What are the differences between seasonal allergic conjunctivitis and acute allergic conjunctivitis?

In essence, it is the rapidity of onset and the absence of the hay fever symptoms that distinguishes acute allergic conjunctivitis from SAC (*Table 5.2*).

TABLE 5.2 Seasonal *versus* acute allergic conjunctivitis	
Seasonal allergic conjunctivitis	**Acute allergic conjunctivitis**
Episodic	Single or sporadic episodes
Young atopic person	Not necessarily atopic
Precipitated by grass pollen	Plant allergen likely
Other hay fever symptoms present	Chemosis dominant symptom
Presents to general practitioner	Presents to eye casualty

5.14 What are the features of vernal keratoconjunctivitis?

Vernal keratoconjunctivitis or vernal catarrh is a rare and serious ocular allergy of childhood which usually presents before the age of 10 (range 3–25) years. This is largely a disease affecting young atopic individuals, and 85% of patients are male. Sufferers frequently have a personal (75%) or family history of allergy. The disorder is recurrent and, as suggested by its name (*vernal* being Latin for spring), it has a seasonal pattern. Symptoms begin in the spring and continue through the summer but, if severe, the condition can be present throughout the year. Spontaneous resolution usually occurs after 5–10 years. This condition is more common in dry, warm countries such as Greece and Italy.

Symptoms consist of intense itching, mild photophobia, stringy discharge, watering and the sensation of a foreign body in the eye. There may also be drooping of the upper lids; this mechanical ptosis is caused by the extensive inflammation beneath the upper lid. A complaint of blurred vision is suggestive of corneal involvement (erosions, ulcers or scarring) and requires specialist assessment as vision may be threatened.

On examination one finds 'cobblestone'-like papillae under the top lid. This inflammation and lumpiness is often confined to the top lid, with the lower lid appearing normal. The eye may be red, with follicles around the edge of the cornea; these are said to resemble grains of rice.

5.15 Is atopic keratoconjunctivitis also a disease of children?

No, this is exclusively a disease of atopic adults. Atopic keratoconjunctivitis (AKC) is a potentially blinding disease and the most serious of all ocular allergic conditions. Fortunately it is rare.

By definition, AKC has a 100% association with atopic disease such as eczema and asthma. It is a disease of young and middle-aged adults (20–50 years) and more commonly affects males. It follows a prolonged and serious course with a high incidence of reduction in vision from corneal involvement such as ulcers and scarring. Conjunctival scarring, severe lid eczema and blepharitis are frequently seen and can cause further corneal damage.

TABLE 5.3 Distinguishing between the two forms of allergic keratoconjunctivitis

Vernal keratoconjunctivitis	Atopic keratoconjunctivitis
Children	Adults
Spring and summer	Perennial
Not always atopic	Atopic individual
Involves upper eyelids	Involves lower conjunctiva
Grumbling	Chronic and severe
Secondary corneal changes may occur	Complications common and severe
Topical treatment	Topical and systemic treatment

5.16 When should one be alerted to the possibility of atopic keratoconjunctivitis in a patient?

When an adult atopic patient complains of symptoms that are similar to vernal keratoconjunctivitis. Symptoms may have a seasonal component but normally occur all year round and consist of intense itching, tearing, burning, heavy mucoid discharge and blurred vision. Clinical signs include redness, loss of lid laxity caused by scarring of the conjunctiva of the lids and corneal involvement (punctate or macro erosions, infected ulcers and neovascularization). A number of patients may have keratoconus and cataracts (10%). See *Table 5.3* for the differential diagnosis of the two types of keratoconjunctivitis.

5.17 What is the allergic eye disorder that contact lens wearers suffer?

This is giant papillary conjunctivitis (GPC). This is caused by a combination of chronic low-grade trauma and a hypersensitivity reaction to a foreign body. It is now most commonly seen in the wearers of contact lenses, but traditionally was seen in patients with artificial eyes and protruding sutures.

The probability of developing GPC during contact lens wear increases with longer wearing time, larger diameter lenses, damaged or scratched lenses and heavy protein deposits on the lens. Therefore the wearers of soft lenses are particularly vulnerable.

Patients complain of itching and burning, watering, blurring of vision and reduced tolerance of their lenses. These symptoms usually precede the clinical signs of giant papillae ('large cobblestones') on the conjunctiva lining the upper lid. The cornea is usually not effected.

Giant papillary conjunctivitis resolves completely and rapidly after removal of the provoking factor. However, most patients prefer to wear their lenses or prostheses and in this case reducing wearing time, better lens hygiene and changing material may help (*see Question 5.26*).

Mast cell stabilizers such as sodium cromoglycate are also beneficial.

5.18   What else should be considered in the differential diagnosis of a red eye in a contact lens wearer?

Whenever a contact lens wearer complains of a red irritated eye that does not improve within a few hours, a corneal ulcer or corneal abrasion is high on the differential. Alternatively, they may have developed a hypersensitivity reaction to preservatives in their storage or cleaning solutions. The patient may have developed a true allergy or may not be rinsing the enzyme off completely before placing the lens in the eye.

5.19   What is keratoconus?

This is a non-inflammatory disorder of the cornea causing visual impairment, particularly myopia and irregular astigmatism. The cornea becomes steepened and thin and, in extreme cases, can assume a conical shape (hence the name).

There is a definite relationship between atopy and keratoconus, with the prevalence of atopic diseases higher in patients than in normal controls. Atopic patients are bothered by itching, and it is thought that excessive eye rubbing may contribute to the development of keratoconus. Interestingly, it has a higher incidence in people with Down's syndrome who, like atopic individuals, tend to be vigorous eye rubbers.

MANAGEMENT

5.20   What is the management of seasonal or perennial allergic conjunctivitis?

History and examination are normally sufficient to identify the trigger factors and diagnosis. Should clarification of the allergic trigger still be required, skin prick testing to airborne allergens (or blood tests for specific IgE) are helpful.

First line treatments are:

- Avoidance of trigger factors
  - Full avoidance is rarely practical, but appropriate use of sunglasses and keeping car windows shut while driving are helpful in reducing pollen exposure.
- Topical or systemic antihistamines, or both
  - Oral antihistamines (see pp. 57–59 for side-effects, formulations and dosage). These are the drug of first choice in treating seasonal allergic conjunctivitis and are particularly useful in reducing itchiness.
  - Topical antihistamines, when combined with a vasoconstricting agent, can be effective in reducing redness.

■ Topical mast cell stabilizers
■ Topical sodium cromoglycate (2% solution; 4% ointment) is useful when symptoms are not controlled by an oral antihistamine. Dosage is 1–2 drops (or ointment) in each eye four times a day.
Other treatments:

■ Corticosteroids
■ Topical corticosteroids are effective but may produce serious side-effects, e.g. glaucoma, exacerbations of herpetic keratitis and corneal thinning. They have no role in the primary care management of allergic conjunctivitis.
■ Oral steroids are used occasionally as short courses and only in patients with very severe symptoms. Oral steroids should only be prescribed under the supervision of an ophthalmologist because of the risk of adverse events and/or misdiagnosis.

5.21 Is there ever a role for immunotherapy?

Immunotherapy is of limited use and should only be considered in those patients with severe seasonal symptoms of allergic conjunctivitis and rhinitis and in whom symptoms are not controlled on conventional drug therapy.

5.22 How does topical sodium cromoglycate work?

Sodium cromoglycate blocks mast cell degranulation in the conjunctiva. It is best used as a prophylactic as it has little effect on established symptoms. Maximum impact is achieved with drops initially four times a day, and then reducing to twice daily. Such an intensive regimen is not always convenient and is particularly impractical for the young school child. Adult patients will often decide for themselves whether the improvement of symptoms achieved is worth the effort invested.

To increase the dosing interval, more viscous preparations have been developed, but these have not been well tolerated.

If a patient seems to be achieving less than optimal control but claims to be compliant it may be worth reviewing their technique for instilling the drops (*see Questions 5.27–5.29*).

5.23 How does one reduce the threat to vision in atopic keratoconjunctivitis?

The mechanism of the disease is complex and not fully understood. As treatment is difficult it requires the help of a specialist ophthalmologist.

Treatment is with anti-inflammatory medication such as sodium cromoglycate eye drops 2% together with symptom relief (cold compress, lubricants or mucus-dissolving agents). Topical steroids are by far the most effective treatment but their use is moderated by the risk of side-effects (*see Question 5.20*). Immunotherapy is of no value.

A newer agent, cyclosporin A (2% ointment or drops), is effective in controlling the disease, but patients complain that it causes stinging on installation.

Treatment of the blepharitis and facial eczema is usually achieved with topical steroids or cyclosporin A as a steroid sparing agent. In severe cases, oral steroids and other immunosuppressive agents may be necessary.

5.24 If a patient with glaucoma develops an allergic reaction to topical medication what is the most likely offender?

Apraclonidine has the highest incidence of allergic reactions, followed by epinephrine, dipivefrin, beta-blockers and pilocarpine. If a patient is taking apraclonidine, timolol and pilocarpine to control their intraocular pressures there are ways round this! A frequently used strategy is to stop the apraclonidine, change the beta-blocker to carteolol (the best tolerated beta-blocker) and to change the pilocarpine to carbachol.

In a patient who takes medication bilaterally there is the potential to conduct a comparative trial by changing the beta-blocker in one eye and the pilocarpine in the other; in this way one should be able to detect which was the offending medication. Similar strategies can be adopted when trying to isolate the offending medication when there is polypharmacy for other conditions.

PROGNOSIS

5.25 What is the prognosis for allergic eye disease?

Allergic conjunctivitis is not a serious or sight-threatening disease, but the various forms of keratoconjunctivitis are serious diseases requiring expert management.

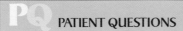 **PATIENT QUESTIONS**

5.26 Having had a problem with giant papillary conjunctivitis is it safe to continue wearing contact lenses?

Lenses should not be worn at all until symptoms settle. Your optometrist will advise you but it is suggested that, if you wish to wear lenses again, you should buy a new pair, be scrupulous about lens hygiene and reduce wearing times. Changing the lens type from soft to gas-permeable may prevent recurrence. It is possible that you are sensitive to the preservative in one of the lens solutions so it may also be worth trying a preservative-free solution if lens wear is tried again.

5.27 What is the best way of inserting eye drops? (*Fig. 5.1*)

Make yourself comfortable, either sitting or lying
Pull down the lower lid to form a 'sac'
Hold the eye drops in your other hand, bring the dropper close to the eye and squeeze one drop into the sac
Close the eye and blot any excess solution with a clean tissue.
See also *Box 5.3*.

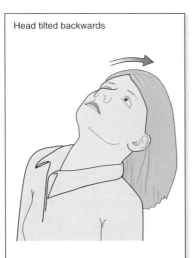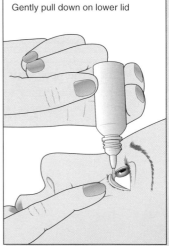

▲

Fig 5.1 Insertion of eye drops.

5.28 Does it matter if I use more than the recommended number of drops?

If more than one drop arrives in your eye by mistake there is no need for any concern because the excess will spill onto your cheek so it is quite difficult to overdose!

5.29 Are there any tricks for getting eye drops into children's eyes?

Some adults don't like having eye drops and so it is understandable that young children may not always be fully cooperative! Rather than battle, it may be better to lie the child down and put a drop into the inner corner of the closed eye. When the child opens their eyes the drop will trickle in. The success of this approach is dependent upon persuading the child to remain lying down until the task is complete.

BOX 5.3 Three important things to remember about eye drops to avoid infections

- ■ Do not allow other people to use your eye drops
- ■ Do not allow the dropper to touch the eye or anything else
- ■ Keep and dispose of the eye drops exactly as instructed on the packaging

---

Anaphylaxis

INTRODUCTION

6.1   What is anaphylaxis?

Anaphylaxis is a multisystem IgE-mediated allergic reaction resulting in hypertension, urticaria, angioedema, asthma, gastrointestinal upset and, sometimes, death. The onset of symptoms occurs within minutes or, on occasion, within seconds after exposure to the responsible allergen.

6.2   Which allergens most commonly cause anaphylaxis and which patients are most at risk?

Penicillin hypersensitivity is the most frequent cause of anaphylaxis, followed by wasp and bee venoms, latex and food allergens (peanuts, other nuts, fish, shellfish and eggs).

In extremely sensitized individuals, even the smell of the relevant allergen may cause anaphylaxis. In this way, nut-allergic patients may be affected in aeroplanes when the little bags of peanuts are opened at cocktail time. The dust from these packets enters the air conditioning system and is recirculated in sufficient concentration to affect those with the highest level of nut sensitivity. Patients with cardiovascular disease and other major disorders are more likely to die from anaphylaxis than those who are otherwise healthy.

In hospital, apart from antibiotics, there are several scenarios which are commonly associated with anaphylaxis. These include blood transfusion, general anaesthesia, local anaesthesia and radiocontrast materials used for certain types of X-ray examination. However, almost any drug can cause allergic reactions in an unlucky patient, especially if given intravenously.

DIAGNOSIS

6.3   How should patients with anaphylaxis be investigated and managed?

All patients with anaphylaxis should be investigated to determine the cause. The mainstay of treatment is avoidance: accurate identification of the offending substance prevents the unnecessary inconvenience of avoiding substances that are in fact harmless.

The following general rules should be followed while waiting for assessment:

■ Avoid exposure to the allergen thought to have caused the reaction.
■ Avoid cross-reacting allergens as well (see *Table 9.1*).

■ Avoid beta-blockers.
■ Train the patient to self-administer adrenaline.

6.4 What tests are useful and relevant?

The most important aspect of diagnosis is to take a comprehensive history, recording separately details of what exactly happened and the opinions of the patients and/or relatives regarding possible causes. Where food or drugs are implicated, note the timing of ingestion of the food or drug in relation to the onset of the episode. Also note whether the food or drug has been tolerated before and/or after the event without any symptoms. Specific investigations should aim at validating the conclusion drawn from the history. Useful tests may include allergy skin tests, blood tests for specific IgE, tests of the complement system, autoantibody screens, biochemical screens, thyroid function tests and, occasionally, formal challenge tests with suspect substances, although the risk:benefit ratio of any such challenges must be carefully assessed.

MANAGEMENT

6.5 How should anaphylaxis be managed in primary care?

If faced with a patient presenting with an anaphylactic reaction, the priority is to bring the current episode under control. Analysis of the causes of the reaction can wait. Life-threatening anaphylaxis should be treated with prompt administration of adrenaline (subcutaneously or intramuscular, never intravenously), as well as giving antihistamines and hydrocortisone. Plasma expanders can be given in hypotensive patients, but they will usually respond to adrenaline.

Once the immediate danger is over, a careful history should be obtained from the patient and any witnesses. Detailed investigation of the causes of the episode should be deferred until the dust has settled. If there is doubt about the cause and nature of the episode, an adrenaline syringe for self-administration should be provided and the patient instructed in its correct use.

6.6 What are the issues to be considered before prescribing a patient self-administered adrenaline?

Adrenaline is a very useful drug for dealing with the acute effects of histamine. However, if given to an otherwise fit individual, it will cause transient hypertension and tachycardia, and has occasionally caused transient ischaemic attacks or even strokes. Prompt use of adrenaline during an anaphylactic episode will abort the attack and will buy 20–30 min to get to hospital and/or obtain medical advice. Adrenaline is indicated for patients who have life-threatening generalized attacks or who have compromise of their airway during an episode. Facial swelling and/or urticaria are not indications in their own right.

6.7 What should you tell a patient prescribed an Epipen?

First and foremost the patient needs to know when to use the Epipen and how to use it. Patients should be reassured that they will not drop dead just because they develop some urticaria or facial swelling, but they need to understand that they should use their pen at the first signs of any compromise to their breathing or if there are other features indicating hypotension. Some patients find it difficult to distinguish this from the natural panic which sets in when they start to develop an anaphylactic event. Such patients may end up using their adrenaline syringe much more often than is really necessary and will need re-educating when they return for their repeat prescription. Any patient given an Epipen needs to be shown how to use the device. This demonstration should, if possible, also be witnessed by their partners/parents/children so that more than one person knows how to use the adrenaline syringe. Patients should be advised to carry the Epipen with them on holiday or when dining out as it is no use in their bathroom cabinet at home when they have an anaphylactic reaction at a picnic or in a restaurant. Patients should be told that it is possible to use an Epipen through clothing and that it is best administered into the outer aspect of the thigh where there are no blood vessels or nerves of any consequence. The patient should also be advised on how to dispose of a used Epipen and on the procedure for obtaining a replacement.

6.8 What instructions should be given on the use of an Epipen?

- Place the Epipen in the palm of your right hand (or left hand if left-handed) with the grey cap towards the thumb.
- Form a fist around the pen.
- With the other hand remove the grey safety cap.
- Place the black tip against the outer thigh (it can be used through clothing).
- Using a quick motion, press against the thigh until the unit activates. (NB. The training unit clicks when it is activated but the actual pen does not click.)
- Remind patients not to put their fingers over the black tip where the needle comes out.
- Do not put thumb over end of unit.
- Do not use the grey safety cap until ready to use. Once removed, the pen will activate whenever the black tip is pushed.

After use, the device should not be placed in household rubbish but taken to a doctor's surgery, pharmacy or hospital for proper safe disposal.

6.9 A patient says they collapsed in the dentist's chair. Could this be an allergy to local anaesthetic and how should this be managed?

The commonest cause of collapse in a dentist's chair is simple vasovagal fainting. However, some patients are allergic to latex and others have genuine reactions to local anaesthetic. Ideally, all such patients should be reviewed by a specialist allergy service which is able to differentiate between these various possibilities. The first step is to get an accurate history of what happened, together with the timing of the episode relative to the drugs that were given. Allergy is more likely if there was a rash or marked local swelling. Any history of latex allergy (reaction to condoms, balloons, etc. or cross-reactions with bananas, chestnuts, tropical fruits, etc.) should be documented. Skin tests can be performed to local anaesthetic, including both those used at the time of the episode and also a number of alternatives that could be used on subsequent occasions if it turns out that the patient is indeed allergic. Tests for latex allergies should be performed at the same time. In over 99% of cases the skin tests will all be negative but, when the tests are positive, they are usually very reliable and the patient should be given written information on the nature of the test that was performed and the advice that has been given. This information should be copied to the dentist and the GP. The patient should also receive a copy to show to any other party involved in their care.

If antibiotics and/or any other medication were given at the same time as the episode, the possibilities of allergy to these drugs should also be considered. Finally, patients with C1 esterase inhibitor deficiency will often experience large local swellings following any form of surgery or manipulations. Dentistry is no exception and so, when there is a clear history of swelling and no obvious explanation after the initial investigation, ask about a possible family history of swellings and consider the possibility of a complement defect.

6.10 What is the optimum treatment for patients with a history of reacting to bee or wasp stings?

Allergy to bee venom is seen mainly in beekeepers, their relatives and neighbours. Allergy to wasp venom is more random, although some occupations are at high risk (greengrocers, bakers, ice-cream sellers, gardeners, etc.). If there is an occupational risk the best management strategy is to reduce the risk. Otherwise, the risk of being re-stung is relatively low and can be further minimized by common sense precautions:

■ Never disturb insect nests or hives.
■ Stay away from areas that attract insects, such as litter bins.

■ Do not walk barefoot out of doors in summer.
■ Wear dull colours (green, khaki) rather than orange or yellow, both of which are highly attractive to wasps.
■ Do not wear loose clothing in which insects can get trapped.

Desensitization should be considered in those who have had life-threatening systemic reactions, and who still have high concentrations of venom-specific IgE. As this form of treatment is time-consuming and not widely available, the decision to desensitize has to include consideration of the practicality of the patient attending for regular injections. An adrenaline pen and antihistamine tablets should be given as a first aid package for anyone who has had a systemic reaction in the past 10 years. This will help to restore the patient's confidence to go out and about, although it is unlikely to have a major impact on mortality rates (because the background fatality rate is so low).

6.11 Do all patients with anaphylaxis have to be referred?

This depends on the level of expertise of the person who sees them. The important thing is that anyone with anaphylaxis should be assessed by somebody who has expertise in the area, understands the issues and can arrange appropriate investigation.

6.12 Why do patients who suffer recurrent anaphylactic attacks and use self-administered adrenaline still need to be seen in Casualty departments?

Up to 20% of patients treated for the initial event will have a further life-threatening event after 6–8 h. Being 'seen in Casualty' of itself is not sufficient, but rather these patients require a period of observation somewhere in which they can be treated in the event of recurrent angioedema or anaphylaxis.

6.13 What is the role of adrenaline inhalers?

Inhaled adrenaline has been used as another means of delivering adrenaline during anaphylaxis. These devices were originally introduced to treat asthma, but have largely been replaced in this role by selective beta-agonists such as salbutamol. CFC-propelled adrenaline inhalers (e.g. Medihaler-epi) were used for many years in people experiencing allergic reactions short of anaphylaxis, and offered a less invasive form of therapy compared to injectable adrenaline. The Medihaler-epi was sprayed into the mouth and absorbed rapidly from under the tongue, and also dealt directly with any bronchospasm. Following the withdrawal of CFC propellants, the

Medihaler-epi was discontinued and there are no plans to develop an adrenaline aerosol using the non-CFC propellants. Water-based adrenaline sprays are available in some markets and can be imported through pharmacies on a named patient basis. However, most patients who used to be prescribed Medihaler-epi have been reassessed and those who genuinely continue to need adrenaline have been offered injectable adrenaline.

Adrenaline inhalers are prescribed to be used with antihistamine tablets and oral corticosteroids (see treatment plan below).

Patients should be told that, as soon as they experience any of the symptoms which suggest they may be getting another severe allergic reaction, they should:

■ Take two puffs of the Medihaler and repeat this dose every 2 min up to a maximum of 20 puffs in 20 min.
■ Take a single dose of antihistamine.
■ Take a single dose of steroid.
■ Continue the antihistamine and steroid tablets for 3 days.

Adrenaline is the drug of first choice in severe anaphylactic reactions, severe airway obstruction, laryngeal oedema, severe urticaria or angioedema. By stimulating alpha-adrenoreceptors it reverses the peripheral vasodilatation observed in oedema and urticaria, and restores blood pressure towards normal. Adrenaline is a beta-agonist and, as such, dilates the airways and suppresses further release of histamine and leukotrienes.

6.14   Can self-administration of adrenaline cause serious side-effects?

Adrenaline is relatively safe. Caution is required with the very elderly and those with cardiac problems. Patients should be reassured that there is little or no risk of harmful effects from a dose of adrenaline that is not strictly necessary, whereas waiting until they are sure the reaction is severe may leave things too late.

Patients must be reminded to check the dose on the adrenaline emergency kit to ensure it is of maximum potency. In the US, there is an Epipen replacement reminder programme: about 1 month before the unit is due to expire the manufacturers send the patient a reminder to contact their doctor for a new prescription. Enrolment forms for the free programme can be found on the patient insert inside every Epipen box.

6.15   What is the role of desensitization in patients who have suffered anaphylaxis?

This depends on the agent that was responsible for the anaphylaxis. Suitable extracts and treatment regimes are available for wasp and bee venoms, but not yet for any of the foods that are associated with anaphylaxis. Drug-induced reactions are best treated by avoidance of the drug, although there is a desensitizing regime for aspirin for use in patients who have to take aspirin on a regular basis (usually patients with severe forms of arthritis who do not tolerate other forms of therapy).

6.16 What is the natural history of anaphylaxis?

In contrast to angioedema and urticaria, anaphylaxis usually has a specific cause. If the trigger can be avoided then the condition will not recur. The natural history therefore depends to a large extent on one's ability to identify the trigger and avoid it. In patients with insect venom anaphylaxis, the likelihood of recurrence on repeat sting is about 50% to start with and declines gradually over time, reaching a background risk (equivalent to that of the general population) after about 10 years.

6.17 Can children grow out of anaphylaxis?

Children with allergy to bee or wasp stings have a good chance, perhaps as high as 50%, of growing out of their allergy. About 20% of children with anaphylaxis to peanut will lose their sensitivity by the age of 18 years, but it is probably safest to assume that the condition will be lifelong.

It is possible to assess the strength of the residual sensitization by radio-allergosorbent test (RAST) or skin prick testing, but this will tend to overestimate rather than underestimate the risk of anaphylaxis. Those with negative tests for specific IgE are safe; those with positive tests may react but will not necessarily do so.

PATIENT QUESTIONS

6.18 If one member of the family is anaphylactic to a foodstuff should the rest of the family avoid eating it?

This is one way of reducing exposure in the home environment but may not be entirely appropriate. For foods where the patient reacts even to the smell of the food or to tiny traces, it makes sense to minimize exposure, but for other foods where it is only digestion of significant amounts that causes a problem then the priority is to take care to avoid cross-contamination of food. Children with allergies need to learn to take responsibility for avoiding their allergens, and this may not be helped by creating an allergy-free environment in the home. Moreover, removal of a favourite item (peanut butter, shrimp, etc.) may create resentment within the family and unnecessary stress between family members.

6.19 What advice should be given to schools where a pupil is anaphylactic?

The school needs to know the degree of sensitivity and whether complete avoidance of the food in the child's environment is essential. If adrenaline has been prescribed, schools need to have access to this and need to have trained members of staff available to administer it. A balance has to be struck between protecting the child with an allergy and allowing those who do not have allergies to lead normal existences. Creating divisions in groups of pupils is not desirable, especially as many older children want to be seen as part of a single peer group. Some confusion has arisen because of conflicting advice given to schools in different areas by different personnel. Most schools now have policies for asthma, but this is not true for other allergic conditions, and so useful and coherent advice and information will often be appreciated, but should always be based on practical and sensible principles.

6.20 Are there any problems carrying Epipens on aircraft?

With the increase in security measures at airports following the terrorist attacks of 11th September 2001, it is possible that patients may experience difficulties getting clearance to carry Epipens on board. Patients should carry a letter from their physician on headed notepaper. The wording of the letter should be along the lines of :

'[Patient's name] suffers from a life-threatening allergy and must carry an Epipen at all times in case of accidental exposure to the allergen. An Epipen is an auto-injector of adrenaline and its use may be life-saving for this person. The prescription of adrenaline is a medical necessity for this person and they must carry the Epipen at all times, including on all airline flights.'

Angioedema and urticaria

7

INTRODUCTION

7.1 What are urticaria and angioedema?

Urticaria (*Fig. 7.1*) means nettle rash (*Urtica* is the Latin name for the stinging nettle). Urticaria can show up as small itchy weals looking like small insect bites or can form large plaques which are raised, red at the edge and often white with slight anaesthesia in the centre. The size and distribution of the weals can vary quite rapidly over time and they do not usually leave any scar. However, the skin may be discoloured, especially after large-scale attacks, and the skin may feel slightly strange when touched. This reflects a mild degree of residual oedema, which affects the nerve endings. Angioedema is caused by a similar process happening just below the skin surface. This causes soft tissue swelling and is most often seen on the face and in the throat. Not only are the tissues in this area quite soft, and so swell up easily, but also we are very aware of small changes in people's faces. Thus even a tiny amount of swelling on the face is noticed whereas a larger amount of swelling on the arm or leg might go unnoticed by the patient or onlookers.

7.2 Do the same mechanisms operate in urticaria and angioedema?

Both conditions involve the activation of specialized skin cells called mast cells, which contain histamine.

Histamine causes weals when injected into the skin and soft tissue oedema when injected subcutaneously. There are some other chemical mediators involved which are also released from the mast cell but, in most patients, the histamine predominates. Allergy is one of the mechanisms that can trigger the mast cell but there are many other ways in which a mast cell can become activated. These include direct effects of drugs (especially opiates), viral infections, antibodies directed against molecules on the mast cell surface, complement

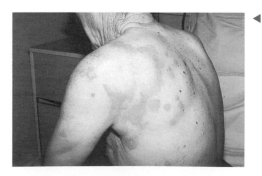

◀ **Fig 7.1** Urticaria.

components (C3a and C5a), several cytokines and chemokines, etc. The critical difference between urticaria and angioedema is the location at which the mast cell activation occurs. That said, complement activation is more likely to cause angioedema than urticaria, presumably because complement activation takes place in soft tissue but is not normally triggered at the skin surface.

7.3 Is histamine the only mediator involved?

No. Although antihistamines will control most episodes of urticaria, other mediators are released in most patients. These include leukotrienes and various mast cell enzymes. From a clinical perspective, this allows a sensible choice of additional or alternative medication if antihistamines fail to bring the condition under control.

7.4 Does urticaria always have an allergic cause? (See *Box 7.1*)

Urticaria is a common condition, affecting 15–20% of the population at some time during their lives. Although commonly perceived to be of allergic aetiology, this is the case in only a very small minority. In most cases urticaria is idiopathic.

DIAGNOSIS

7.5 How should patients with urticaria be investigated and managed?

An accurate history is essential. It is important to distinguish between patients in whom urticaria is the sole symptom, and those in whom urticaria is part of a more generalized allergic reaction (*Question 6.1*).

BOX 7.1 Causes of urticaria

Allergens such as bee and wasp stings, food (especially fruits, shellfish, nuts and dairy products), and drugs such as penicillin
Non-allergic causes include:
  Physical causes (pressure, temperature change)
  Painkillers and anti-inflammatory drugs (common culprits are ibuprofen, aspirin, paracetamol and opioid analgesics)
  Virus infections
  Some food dyes, such as tartrazine (E number 102) and food preservatives (ascorbic acid, sulphites, antioxidants)
Rarer causes include vasculitic disorders, blood products, radiocontrast media, hepatitis B and hereditary angioedema (see below)

7.6 What tests are useful and relevant?

The most important aspect of diagnosis is to take a comprehensive history, recording separately details of what exactly happened and the opinions of the patients and/or relatives regarding possible causes. Where food or drugs are implicated, note the timing of ingestion of the food or drug in relation to the onset of the episode. Also note whether the food or drug has been tolerated before and/or after the event without any symptoms. Specific investigations will be aimed at validating the conclusion drawn from the history. Useful tests include allergy skin tests, blood tests for specific IgE, tests of the complement system, autoantibody screens, biochemical screens, thyroid function tests and, occasionally, formal challenge tests with suspect substances, although the risk:benefit ratio of any such challenges must be carefully assessed.

7.7 Can drug allergy be accurately diagnosed?

Drug allergy is one of the potential causes of anaphylaxis, angioedema and urticaria, and should always be considered when a patient presents with these conditions. A detailed history of the episodes and their relationship to the ingestion of medication will help to indicate whether there is a possible link. Drugs which have been taken regularly without adverse reactions are most unlikely to be responsible. To be relevant, the drug should have been ingested within a few hours of the onset of the episode, or else have a clear and recurrent link to a series of episodes. Drugs which have been tolerated on subsequent occasions are also unlikely to have been responsible.

Specific tests for drug allergies are available for penicillins. Reliable skin tests can be performed for local and general anaesthetics, including muscle relaxants. Skin tests can also be undertaken on an *ad hoc* basis for many other drugs, although the reliability of such skin tests has not necessarily been validated.

7.8 How should one investigate a patient complaining of recurrent lip swelling?

Take a careful history of the episodes, including the timing of ingestion of any food or drugs, especially aspirin and other NSAIDs. Investigate for allergy if this seems plausible; otherwise, exclude C1 esterase deficiency, alcoholism, hypothyroidism and autoimmunity. In the absence of these, proceed with symptomatic management (see below).

7.9 Are there any non-specific triggers of urticaria/angioedema?

Viral infections are the commonest cause of recurrent acute urticaria. Some drugs, notably aspirin, can trigger urticaria and angioedema even though they were not the primary cause. Alcohol, exercise and spicy food have also been implicated. The basis of this seems to be that the mast cells are fragile during and after an episode, and it only takes a relatively minor insult to set them off again. Once the condition has settled down, the non-specific triggering should stop.

MANAGEMENT

7.10 Which drug should be tried first for urticaria?

 Assuming that remediable causes have been addressed and dealt with, the management of urticaria is focused on containing symptoms and allowing the mast cells to settle down and return to normal. Suppression of weals seems to accelerate the return to normality so, with the exception of those with very infrequent attacks, it is sensible to try to suppress the rashes. Most urticaria will be fully controlled with an antihistamine. Long-acting non-sedating antihistamines should be used. Desloratadine, cetirizine and fexofenadine are all effective but, if the dose has to be pushed, desloratadine is both the most powerful and the least likely to cause adverse effects when used above standard dosages. Older antihistamines such as chlorpheniramine and hydroxyzine should not be used as they cause unacceptable levels of sedation, even in those who do not think they are affected.

7.11 What does one do next if antihistamines are not fully effective?

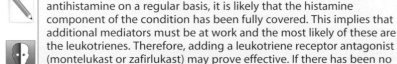

Assuming that the patient has taken a long-acting non-sedating antihistamine on a regular basis, it is likely that the histamine component of the condition has been fully covered. This implies that additional mediators must be at work and the most likely of these are the leukotrienes. Therefore, adding a leukotriene receptor antagonist (montelukast or zafirlukast) may prove effective. If there has been no benefit after 1 month, it is worth trying tranexamic acid 1g b.d. instead of the leukotriene receptor antagonist. The antihistamines should be continued throughout.

Other options which sometimes work include the use of a long-acting beta-adrenoceptor agonist (e.g. bambuterol) which opposes the pharmacological actions of the histamines and also stabilizes mast cells. Oral steroids may be effective in the short term but do not provide lasting benefit. Moreover, their side-effects are unacceptable when used in any way other than short courses. Anabolic steroids such as danazol or stanozolol (no longer listed in *BNF* but still available as a specialist import) can be used to increase the production of C1 esterase inhibitor. These are licensed for use in hereditary angioedema and have sometimes been tried in sporadic antihistamine-resistant angioedema. However, these drugs have significant androgenic potential, inducing virilization and hirsutism in females. Tranexamic acid often works just as well and is much less likely to cause side-effects.

PROGNOSIS

7.12 What is the natural history of urticaria?

The commonest form of urticaria is acute, viral-induced urticaria which may present as a single episode or as a series of brief episodes over a 3–6-week period. Chronic idiopathic urticaria tends to occur every day or several days per week and may continue for 6–18 months before resolving spontaneously. Forms of urticaria which are caused by allergy or other conditions will follow the natural history of the underlying condition. Treatment with anti-allergic drugs seems to accelerate the process of recovery in chronic urticaria, possibly by allowing the mast cells to restabilize. There are histamine receptors on mast cells, lymphocytes and nerve endings which may contribute to the maintenance of urticaria. Hence blocking the effects of histamine should allow a reduction in the degree of mast cell activation, allowing the condition to settle.

7.13 What is the natural history of angioedema?

Like urticaria, the natural history depends on the cause. If there is a specific cause for angioedema then the natural history will follow the course of the underlying condition. If allergies and underlying conditions have been excluded, the natural history is for episodic recurrences which will usually disappear over a period of months, but some patients will experience intermittent episodes over the years. There is nothing about the initial presentation that gives any guide to the likely long-term prognosis.

THE FUTURE

7.14 Are there likely to be new forms of specific immunotherapy for such allergies as peanut and latex?

Research is ongoing to develop vaccines for food allergy and latex allergy. However, at present, no suitable vaccine has been developed that can be used in routine clinical practice. There is also interest in the development of non-specific immunodulatory treatments which might downregulate allergy in general as opposed to being specifically targeted against one food.

PATIENT QUESTIONS

7.15 If one member of the family is allergic to a foodstuff should the rest of the family avoid eating it?

See Question 6.18.

7.16 If my urticaria and angioedema is not due to allergy then what is causing it?

Although many patients understandably think that their rash must be due to something they ate, the reality is that only a small proportion of urticaria and angioedema is caused by food allergy. Some cases are due to drug reactions, and some are due to contact sensitivity (e.g. latex rubber, irritant plants, or chemicals used in the workplace). One type of angioedema runs in families and is due to low levels of a protein involved in switching off immune reactions. A small number are due to overactivity of the immune system, where the body reacts against its own cells, and some are linked to other conditions such as an underactive thyroid gland or liver disease. In over 85% of cases no specific cause will be found. Doctors believe that most of these are probably triggered by viral infections. The viral infection does not have to be very severe, and in some cases it may not cause any symptoms at all, until the urticarial rash appears. Fortunately, if no allergic cause is found and you do not have any of the rare immune system or metabolic conditions that cause angioedema/urticaria, then the natural history is for the rash to settle down gradually over a few weeks or months. Treatment with antihistamines may help to accelerate this process.

Eczema and dermatitis

8

INTRODUCTION

8.1 What is atopic dermatitis?

Atopic dermatitis (often called atopic eczema in the UK) is an inflammatory condition of the skin, characterized by dryness and marked itching. Most of the clinical features are caused by scratching the affected areas. In infancy, the face, scalp and extensor surfaces are affected, but in children over 1 year, the main areas affected are flexural creases and adjacent areas. Sometimes only the hands are affected, with small blister-like lesions called pompholyx.

8.2 What is the difference between eczema and dermatitis?

The nomenclature of skin disorders can appear unnecessarily confusing because of the tendency to use shorthand terms. The term dermatitis simply means 'inflammation of the skin' and can be correctly applied to a number of conditions. In medical use, atopic dermatitis is the form of dermatitis associated with IgE antibodies, asthma and rhinitis, in which there are usually no external triggers. Allergic contact dermatitis is caused by sensitization to external agents, typically chemicals. In common parlance, dermatitis is used as shorthand for allergic contact dermatitis and atopic dermatitis is referred to as eczema.

8.3 How important is allergy in causing atopic dermatitis and contact dermatitis?

Allergic contact dermatitis is always caused by an allergic reaction to an external agent (see below).

This type of allergic response involves lymphocytes rather than antibodies (i.e. it is a form of cell-mediated hypersensitivity). In childhood eczema, there is good evidence that ingestion of egg and cow's milk can trigger exacerbations of eczema, although the precise mechanisms involved are uncertain. The role of allergy in adult eczema is less clearly defined. Many patients with atopic eczema have very high concentrations of total IgE and, in many such patients, there are high concentrations of IgE directed against house dust mite.

Dermatitis can also be caused by irritants without requiring specific allergic sensitization. Agents incriminated in irritant/occupational dermatitis include acids, alkalis, cutting oils, detergents and solvents. In high concentrations these agents may cause chemical burns and ulceration, but at lower levels of exposure, exposed skin reacts with a picture that can be difficult to distinguish from allergic contact dermatitis. However, there will be a history of exposure to irritants, and negative patch tests to contact allergens.

8.4   Which allergens are commonly involved in causing contact dermatitis?

A wide range of chemicals and proteins can cause contact dermatitis (*Box 8.1*). Elastoplast, nickel (especially jewellery and studs on jeans) and lanolin (in wool) are the commonest sensitivities in the general population. The prevalence of nickel allergy rises sharply in girls between the ages of 12 and 16, when wearing of jewellery becomes commonplace. In former times it was the nickel in suspender fastenings for stockings and not the nickel in ear-rings that was the commonest cause of nickel allergy! Sensitizing chemicals are also encountered in many occupational settings, including epoxy resins, rubber gloves and chemicals used in hairdressing.

BOX 8.1 Common environmental allergens causing allergic contact dermatitis

Nickel
Cobalt
Rubber accelerators
Fragrances
Chrome
Formaldehyde
Medicaments (neomycin, preservatives)
Adhesives
Epoxy resins
Plastics
Dyes
Plants

8.5   Does the site of inflammation give a clue to the sensitizer?

Yes, very much so. *Figure 8.1* may help to track down the offending substance.

8.6   Which occupations are at greatest risk of contact dermatitis?

Hairdressers are the most at risk, with 120 new cases per 100 000 workers per year. Printers, machine tool operators, car assemblers, machine tool setters, bricklayers, carpenters and people working in the gas and petroleum industry are also at substantially increased risk.

8.7   What is the role of house dust mite in eczema?

Many patients with atopic eczema are sensitized to house dust mite, and this has generally been regarded as an incidental feature. However, a clinical

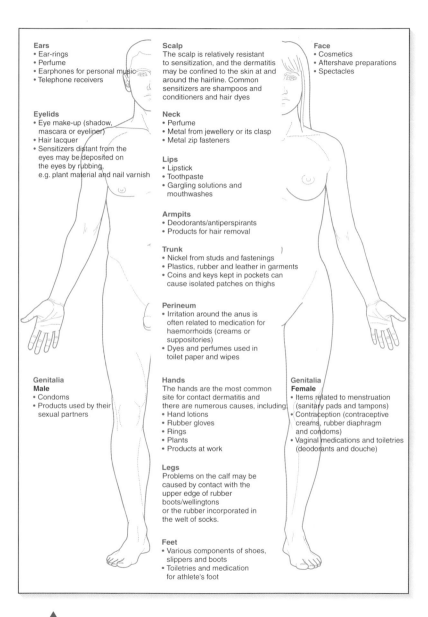

Ears
- Ear-rings
- Perfume
- Earphones for personal music
- Telephone receivers

Eyelids
- Eye make-up (shadow, mascara or eyeliner)
- Hair lacquer
- Sensitizers distant from the eyes may be deposited on the eyes by rubbing, e.g. plant material and nail varnish

Scalp
The scalp is relatively resistant to sensitization, and the dermatitis may be confined to the skin at and around the hairline. Common sensitizers are shampoos and conditioners and hair dyes

Neck
- Perfume
- Metal from jewellery or its clasp
- Metal zip fasteners

Lips
- Lipstick
- Toothpaste
- Gargling solutions and mouthwashes

Armpits
- Deodorants/antiperspirants
- Products for hair removal

Trunk
- Nickel from studs and fastenings
- Plastics, rubber and leather in garments
- Coins and keys kept in pockets can cause isolated patches on thighs

Perineum
- Irritation around the anus is often related to medication for haemorrhoids (creams or suppositories)
- Dyes and perfumes used in toilet paper and wipes

Face
- Cosmetics
- Aftershave preparations
- Spectacles

Genitalia
Male
- Condoms
- Products used by their sexual partners

Hands
The hands are the most common site for contact dermatitis and there are numerous causes, including:
- Hand lotions
- Rubber gloves
- Rings
- Plants
- Products at work

Legs
Problems on the calf may be caused by contact with the upper edge of rubber boots/wellingtons or the rubber incorporated in the welt of socks.

Feet
- Various components of shoes, slippers and boots
- Toiletries and medication for athlete's foot

Genitalia
Female
- Items related to menstruation (sanitary pads and tampons)
- Contraception (contraceptive creams, rubber diaphragm and condoms)
- Vaginal medications and toiletries (deodorants and douche)

Fig 8.1 Common sites and sensitizers.

trial of house dust mite allergen avoidance has shown some benefits in the management of eczema. This suggests that contact allergy to house dust mite may play a part in the pathogenesis of the disease.

DIAGNOSIS

8.8 Are there criteria for diagnosing eczema?

The initial diagnosis remains clinical, based on history and features. For clinical purposes, patients must have an itchy skin condition (this may present as scratching or rubbing in a child), plus at least three of the following features:

- Itching in flexures (or on cheeks in child less than 4 years)
- History of atopy (or an atopic first-degree relative in a child less than 4 years)
- General tendency to dry skin in previous year
- Visible flexural eczema (or on the cheeks, forehead or limbs of children under 4 years)
- Onset in the first 2 years of life.

More rigorous lists of diagnostic criteria (e.g. the Hanifin and Risjka criteria) are used to identify atopic dermatitis patients for inclusion in clinical trials, but those listed above suffice for standard clinical practice.

8.9 How can one test for allergic causes of eczema?

Allergic contact dermatitis can be confirmed by patch testing (see below).

8.10 Is food allergy relevant in eczema?

Food allergy does seem to play a role in young children with eczema. In particular, allergy to egg and cow's milk are common in eczematous children under 2 years of age, and can be shown to be clinically relevant by improvement on elimination, followed by exacerbation on reintroduction. However, there are many eczematous children and adults who have positive skin tests to food allergens without any clinical symptoms associated with ingestion of the relevant foods. In other words, false-positive immediate skin tests are common, and may reflect a general, polyclonal stimulation of IgE production rather than clinically important specific sensitivities.

8.11 What key features distinguish atopic dermatitis from allergic contact dermatitis?

Allergic contact dermatitis is unusual in children and the elderly. The parts of the body affected are limited to those that have come in contact with the causal allergen.

8.12   I have a patient who has been labelled as having intrinsic atopic dermatitis; what is this?

Intrinsic atopic dermatitis is used to describe a subgroup of patients with atopic dermatitis who have normal serum total IgE levels, undetectable allergen-specific IgE levels (measured by radioallergosorbent test, Phadiotop® or CAP® systems), and negative skin prick test towards allergens. But, as in atopic dermatitis, T cells largely infiltrate the skin lesions.

8.13   How is patch testing performed?

The test involves placing a series of substances on the skin and leaving them in place for 48 h. The precise technique varies from centre to centre, but experience is essential for correct interpretation. Allergen is applied in aluminium Finn chambers (a disc with a rim) to the patient's skin, usually the back. Allergens can be applied in an inert vehicle such as petroleum jelly or in an aqueous solution. Substances in petroleum jelly are applied directly to the disc solution or on filter paper. The chambers are held in place with non-allergenic tape (Micropore® or equivalent) and left for 48 h. During this time the patient is instructed to keep the area dry and not to remove or tamper with the tests. Bathing and showering should be avoided until after the final reading. After 48 h the tape is removed and the skin is examined for redness and swelling. Some centres would re-examine the skin at 72 and 96 h if there is no reaction at 48 h.

Most centres use a standard series of the most frequent allergens for all patients and put in additional allergen groups according to the patient's clinical history and occupation.

8.14   Who should be patch-tested?

Clinical features may be insufficient to distinguish allergic contact dermatitis from irritant and endogenous eczema. Patch testing is therefore indicated in any patient with:

- Treatment-resistant dermatitis
- Hand dermatitis
- Stasis dermatitis
- Suspected allergy to topical medicaments (e.g. otitis externa)
- Eczema with an unusual distribution
- Suspected occupational contact dermatitis.

8.15   Is patch testing a quantitative or qualitative test?

Patch test results are given in a semiquantitative scale and are usually reported on a three point scale (+, ++, +++). In addition, toxic/irritant reactions and questionable results are documented.

Semi-quantitative scale for patch test results:

- ■ + erythema and minimal palpable infiltration
- ■ ++ erythema and papulation
- ■ +++ erythema, papulation and blister formation.

8.16 How reliable are patch test results?

To avoid false-negative results all anti-inflammatory medications (apart from oral antihistamines) and all corticosteroid ointments at other sites must be discontinued. The recommended discontinuation times are shown below in *Table 8.1*.

To avoid false-positive results, patch tests should not be applied if there are eczematous skin lesions elsewhere on the body. This frequently leads to multiple non-specific test reactions which are not reproducible if re-tested. If positive reactions toward five allergen groups are observed, an 'angry back' is diagnosed and the test results discarded.

8.17 Is the timing of the readings important?

Irritant toxic reactions tend to decrease in strength from 24 to 72 h, whereas truly allergic reactions are stable or may increase in strength. Some allergens require reading at later time points, e.g. antibiotics and corticosteroids may not become positive until day 7 and will look completely negative at day 3.

8.18 A patient has described a 'patch test' on her arm — are there other ways of patch testing?

Both patients and doctors may confuse patch tests with skin prick tests, which are normally performed on the arm in the UK, although they can also be performed on the back (as routinely done in the US). However, it is possible to patch test on the arm, and this may be preferred for substances that are too irritant to apply for the full 48 h. The patient can be asked to report back daily, or to remove the test if the itching becomes too severe.

8.19 Are there any risks to patch testing?

In theory, there is a risk of inducing contact dermatitis to substances to which the patient is not currently sensitized. In all other respects it is a

TABLE 8.1 Recommended discontinuation times for anti-allergic drugs before patch testing

Corticosteroid ointment at test site	1 week
Long-term systemic steroids (>2 weeks' continuous use)	3 weeks
Short-term systemic steroids (20 mg prednisolone/day or more)	1 week
Short-term systemic steroids (<20 mg prednisolone/day)	3 days
Intensive sun exposure	3 weeks

relatively simple, safe and cheap test to perform. Itching or blistering may develop as a response to the test allergens, but will resolve within a few days.

Interpretation of the results is not easy and requires a thorough knowledge of the allergy history and the materials in question. Almost 10% of the normal population with no skin disease will demonstrate unexpected, apparently irrelevant, positive results. This may lead to inappropriate advice being given.

MANAGEMENT

8.20 Is the treatment of atopic dermatitis and allergic contact dermatitis the same?

No. Atopic eczema has to be managed by the regular and long-term use of emollients and topical steroid preparations. For allergic dermatitis, however, treatment may not be necessary if the allergen can be identified and avoided.

8.21 Does immunotherapy have a role in the management of eczema?

Because we are uncertain about the role of specific allergic sensitization in eczema, most doctors agree that specific desensitization is not an appropriate way of treating eczema. Some anecdotal evidence from individual patients suggests that immunotherapy may help in some cases but, as this is a condition which improves and deteriorates without any obvious cause, it is necessary to be cautious about interpreting such uncontrolled reports.

8.22 How can one prevent contact dermatitis?

The main action is to protect the skin from irritants, of which the most common are soaps and detergents. In the workplace, other irritants such as oils and coolants, alkalis, acids and solvents may be important. Non-irritating alternatives (e.g. soap substitutes) should be provided. Gloves are useful, especially for washing up and other household tasks. For preference, they should be worn with a cotton liner, or over a separate pair of cotton gloves.

8.23 Which treatments for eczema are available to the primary care physician?

First-line therapies available for primary care use include emollients, topical steroids, antihistamines, antibiotics and tar preparations.

Second-line therapies that should be used only with advice from specialists include phototherapy, photochemotherapy, immunosuppressant drugs (oral steroids, cyclosporin, azathioprine, methotrexate, cyclophosphamide) and topical immunomodulators (tacrolimus ointment, cyclosporin microemulsion, ascomycin macrolactam). Advice on these agents includes confirmation of the diagnosis and that first-line agents have been appropriately used, as well as specific issues surrounding toxicity and appropriate use of the second-line agent.

8.24   What role do emollients play in the treatment of eczema?

Emollients have an important role to play in the treatment of atopic dermatitis: they form the mainstay of treatment in patients with mild disease and help to reduce the amount of topical steroid used in the maintenance phase of more severe disease. Emollients help to restore the epidermal barrier and so prevent penetration of irritants and allergens. There is also some evidence that they have an anti-inflammatory effect in the skin. However, emollients are generally underused by patients and physicians, both of whom often perceive a greater benefit from steroid preparations.

Emollients are manufactured in water-based and fatty-based forms (creams and ointments, respectively). The water-based formulations are easier to use but less potent, while the fatty-based ones are more effective but less easy to use. Patient preference is extremely important, because the best emollient for the patient is the one that is used frequently and liberally! Older children and adult patients should be given the opportunity to experiment with a number of different preparations and identify the one that suits them best.

8.25   How should emollients be used?

Emollients should be used in three ways: directly on the skin, as a bath oil and as a soap substitute.

Emollients to be used directly on the affected skin

These should be applied three to four times daily, including after bathing, on to moist skin. Adequate amounts should be prescribed and patients encouraged to use them liberally.

Emollients in the bath

Emollient bath oils leave a lipid layer on the skin. One disadvantage is that they also leave a slippery layer in the bath, to which other family members may object. There is a need to be cautious when bathing to prevent falls. Bath oils with additives can be useful in certain circumstances, e.g. antipruritic and antibacterial.

Soap substitute

Normal soaps and so-called moisturizing soaps should be avoided in eczema as they contain surfactants or solvents which strip epidermal lipids from the skin, exacerbating problems of dryness. Instead, patients should be instructed to mix the emollient with a little warm water and use in the same manner as soap.

8.26 How much cream or ointment should be prescribed to eczematous patients?

More than you may think. The tendency for GPs to under prescribe and for patients to underestimate how much to use goes much of the way toward explaining the failure to maximize the benefit of such treatment regimes.

As a rule of thumb, the treatment of extensive eczema requires 500 g each week in an adult and 250 g in a child.

8.27 How should patients be guided in the use of topical steroids?

With emollients the message is about generous use; however, with steroid creams there is a need for closer monitoring. There is an easy way of calculating the amount needed, called the 'Finger Tip Unit' or FTU. An FTU describes the amount of cream dispensed from a standard tube nozzle (5 mm diameter) between the distal finger crease and the top of the finger (this is a similar distance in all fingers, but it is probably simplest to use the index finger). This equates to approximately 0.4–0.5 g of cream. The number of FTUs required to cover the body are shown in *Table 8.2*. Note that for children the dose has to be adjusted with age.

8.28 Are antibiotics ever useful in treating eczema?

Yes. Oral antibiotics are useful for treating the exacerbations of eczema due to infection. Superantigen producing strains of *Staphylococcus aureus* can recruit large numbers of T cells into the skin, promoting inflammation. A *S. aureus* infection should be considered when eczema suddenly worsens and becomes weepy, crusty, pustular or cellulitic. A 10–14-day course of flucloxacillin (or erythromycin in penicillin-sensitive patients) is needed.

TABLE 8.2 Number of 'Finger Tip Units' required to cover body	
One hand	1 FTU
One arm	1 FTU
One foot	2 FTU
One leg	6 FTU
Face and neck	2.5 FTU
Anterior trunk	7 FTU
Posterior trunk	7 FTU
Infant under 1 year	0.25 adult amount
Child 1–4 years	0.33 adult amount
Child 6–10 years	0.5 adult amount

Should the infection be unresponsive then it is necessary to take swabs to exclude methicillin-resistant *S. aureus* or beta-haemolytic *Streptococcus* spp.

A short course of topical steroid and antibacterial combination ointments can be effective when infection is limited to a specific site.

8.29 What are the roles of antihistamines in the first-line treatment of eczema?

The sedative effects of antihistamines can be useful in reducing scratching, but it is more questionable whether histamine actually plays a part in the expression of the disease. Consequently, non-sedating antihistamines have no real place in eczema unless there is associated urticaria.

8.30 Do tar preparations still have a role?

Tar is an antipruritic agent but is rarely used in primary care now as it can be irritating, and concerns about potential carcinogenicity have meant it is no longer prescribable in some EC countries. However, tar bandages are still used in treating lichenified eczema and areas of prurigo.

8.31 What should be avoided in people with a latex allergy?

Most eczematous reactions to rubber gloves are caused by the chemicals used to stabilize rubber rather than the latex itself. People with contact allergy to rubber often experience problems with elastic in underwear, rubber in shoes, etc (*Question 9.10*).

8.32 What should be avoided in people with a lanolin allergy?

Lanolin is present in all woollen clothing, and is also used in a wide range of creams and ointments.

8.33 Which cases require referral to a specialist?

Most cases of mild and moderate eczema can be managed in primary care, but referral to a specialist becomes necessary when:

- Treatment fails
- Requirement for topical steroids is excessive
- Secondary infection, e.g. with Herpes simplex (eczema herpeticum) or bacteria
- Dietary factors are suspected
- Allergen avoidance is being considered.

PROGNOSIS

8.34 What is the natural history of atopic dermatitis?

About 10% of children and 1% of adults have atopic dermatitis. The problem usually becomes less severe during adolescence and may be completely outgrown around puberty. Subsequently the majority of these patients will remain asymptomatic, apart from hand dermatitis caused by contact with irritants such as detergents and oils.

A minority of patients may experience a relapse of their eczema around the age of 20 years. The mechanism for this is not known, but it has been postulated that it may be linked with infection with infectious mononucleosis causing immunomodulation.

If atopic dermatitis continues into adulthood it is commonly 'outgrown' at the menopause in women. For those rare individuals for whom atopic dermatitis continues into old age, the clinical picture tends to be of severe and widespread disease.

8.35 Is the prognosis for atopic dermatitis and allergic contact dermatitis similar?

Atopic dermatitis tends to be at its worst in childhood, and often resolves during adolescence. In those whose atopic dermatitis persists into adulthood, the condition may relapse and remit, and will generally diminish beyond the age of 30 years. The prognosis for allergic contact dermatitis varies with the cause and how easy it is to avoid. If the allergen is something that is unusual and easily avoided (e.g. nail varnish, topical neomycin), complete resolution of the problem can be achieved. However, if the allergen is common in the environment (e.g. nickel or rubber) then avoidance is more difficult and the patient may have a problem for life.

THE FUTURE

8.36 My management of eczema has not seemed to change for many years. Are there any new treatments coming on line?

Topical immunomodulators, e.g. tacrolimus, are an exciting new form of therapy that are effective in eczema with few side-effects. Immunomodulators work in a number of ways: they reduce the number of inflammatory cytokines produced, they downregulate the expression of high affinity IgE receptors, and they reduce inflammatory mediator release from mast cells and basophils.

Tacrolimus is now licensed in the UK for children over 2 years of age. In practice, it is prescribed by dermatologists as it is suggested that it should only be prescribed by those experienced in managing eczema and immunomodulatory therapies. If its safety record is maintained it may enter the primary care armamentarium in the future. Because the skin immune system repairs DNA damage induced by sunlight, there is a theoretical risk of DNA damage and future skin cancer if care is not taken. Patients should be advised to keep out of the sun and to use a high-performance sunblock.

From the initial safety information available, tacrolimus has few side-effects. The main one is a burning sensation and pruritus, which tends to settle after about a week of treatment. Its main advantage is that it does not affect collagen synthesis or cause skin thinning, so it can be used on the face. In addition, it is advantageous for patients with brown or black skin where postinflammatory pigment change is a problem.

PATIENT QUESTIONS

8.37 My child's eczema is always worse after swimming. Should I stop them swimming?

On balance, no, but you can take steps to reduce the deleterious impact of swimming.

■ Where possible, swim in sea or pools where the chlorine levels are not too high
■ Shower after swimming using usual soap substitute
■ Moisturize skin with emollient while still wet and before getting dressed.

When children are swimming during school the teaching staff may need to be made aware of this routine and its importance, because they may need to allow additional time for thorough showering and creaming.

8.38 How common is allergy to condoms?

Some 'allergies' to condoms are excuses! However, irritation caused by the condom or lubricant is not uncommon and a few people do experience a true allergy to the rubber. Rubber allergy does not exclude the use of a condom as plastic condoms are marketed (e.g. Avanti®). These are as well lubricated, thin and as strong as conventional condoms.

8.39 Would my metal allergy contraindicate the use of an intrauterine contraceptive device?

IUDs contain copper, which is rarely the cause of a metal allergy. Most contact allergies to metal bangles and rings are due to nickel. However, copper IUDs have been reported to cause systemic problems (urticaria, angioneurotic oedema) and local reactions (vaginal discharge) when fitted in a person with a true copper allergy. If you report your concerns to your GP or Family Planning doctor, they can arrange for a special patch allergy test if appropriate.

8.40 I have sometimes experienced contact dermatitis after being in the garden. What can I do?

A number of plants can cause contact dermatitis (see *Box 8.2*), particularly chrysanthemums and other members of the daisy family, so choose your plants carefully. Since 1995 all plants on sale are labelled if they can cause skin allergy, but you may have to look very carefully to find this information.

Additional precautions would be always to wear gloves, avoid rubbing your eyes and face and do not use a strimmer as this can spray sap and fibre over your skin.

> **BOX 8.2 Dermatitis after gardening — common culprits in the garden**
>
> *Alstroemeria*
> Chrysanthemum and other members of the daisy family
> *Daphne* — some species
> Ivy
> *Cupressus leylandii*
> *Primula obconica*
> *Schefflera*
> Bulbs of tulips, lilies, hyacinths and narcissi

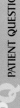

Food allergy

INTRODUCTION

9.1 What sort of adverse reactions can occur to food?

Toxic food reactions will affect anyone exposed to a sufficient amount of food, e.g.

■ chemicals and proteins that occur naturally in the food (e.g. lectins in uncooked kidney beans)
■ contaminants
  ■ fermentation of the foodstuff (e.g. decarboxylation of histidine to form histamine in tuna, salami, etc.)
  ■ inadvertent contamination of the food by deliberate or accidental additions (e.g. staphylococcal toxin in ice cream, ergot in wheat, etc.)

Non-toxic food reactions only occur in certain susceptible individuals and include antibody-driven food allergies, cell-mediated reactions, enzymatic and pharmacological responses, together with a number of reactions that are predictable in individuals, but have unexplained mechanism(s).

9.2 What is food allergy?

Various allergic disorders can be triggered by food. In this sense, food allergy is not really a disease in itself, but a trigger for other clinical conditions. In recent years, food allergy has been blamed for a wide range of symptoms and problems which have little to do with either the immune system or with food. This has led to confusion and doubt about the true nature and extent of food allergy. True food allergy exists and is important, but many people who think they may be allergic to foods may either have a form of food intolerance or have conditions that are unrelated to food.

9.3 What is food sensitivity?

Food sensitivity is an umbrella term which includes any form of adverse reactions to food, including allergic reactions, food intolerance and psychological reactions to food.

9.4 What is the difference between food allergy and food intolerance?

In contrast to food allergy, food intolerances are caused by non-immunological mechanisms following the ingestion of food. Food intolerances may be caused by toxic components of food (histamine in tuna, salmon, etc.), other biogenic amines (migraine after eating cheese, wine, chocolate, etc.), pharmacological properties of the food (e.g. non-specific triggering of histamine release) or symptoms driven by the incomplete digestion of food (e.g. bloating and wind after wheat).

9.5 Does the term food aversion mean the same as food intolerance?

No. Food aversion is when someone dislikes a food, perhaps because they were ill with it once, but there is no evidence of any form of physical adverse reactions when they eat the food. In food intolerance the adverse reaction is reproducible even when the food is given in a disguised form.

9.6 What symptoms may be caused by food allergy?

Many different allergic symptoms can be triggered by food allergy, including:

- Skin reactions: measles-like itchy rashes, eczema, acute urticaria and angioedema. Food allergy is rarely responsible for chronic urticaria.
- Gastrointestinal symptoms: nausea, vomiting, abdominal pain and cramping. Diarrhoea is less frequent.
- Respiratory symptoms: asthma and allergic rhinitis are relatively less common. When caused by food allergy, they usually occur in association with skin and/or gastrointestinal symptoms and are seldom, if ever, an isolated manifestation.

9.7 How can I tell the difference between allergic and toxic reactions to tuna?

Tuna flesh contains large amounts of the amino acid histidine. If fresh tuna is allowed to stand for any length of time before freezing, the histidine can be decarboxylated to form histamine. Once formed, histamine is very stable and is not destroyed by cooking. When eaten, histamine is rapidly absorbed and causes a typical reaction, in which the patient flushes bright red and develops wheezing, tachycardia, hypotension and usually acute diarrhoea. The sufferer feels as if something awful is about to happen — this is a pharmacological effect of histamine on the brain and is in addition to the evidence that something awful is happening! Characteristically, there is no urticaria and little or no perioral swelling (an important distinction from true food allergy which usually causes both). The toxic food reaction is called scombrotoxic food poisoning after the name of the family to which tuna belongs, the Scombridae. Most patients need to be reassured that they do not have a true food allergy before they will contemplate eating tuna again. This can be shown by negative skin prick test or blood test for specific IgE if a verbal explanation if not sufficient to reassure the patient.

NB. The histamine formation can be quite patchy, and people can be completely unaffected despite eating pieces of the fish cut from the flesh adjacent to that eaten by the victim.

9.8 How common is true food allergy?

> True food allergy is driven by IgE antibodies and produces an allergic reaction every time the food is eaten, even in very small amounts. It is, however, relatively rare. Fewer than 5% of children and 1% of adults suffer from true food allergy.

In a large questionnaire survey in the UK almost 10% of the population reported that at some time in their life they had had an unpleasant reaction to food and 5% had reacted to a food additive. When formally challenged to the suspected foodstuffs fewer than 1% of those reporting problems had any reaction at all.

9.9 What are the most likely foods to cause allergic reactions?

In early childhood, egg and cow's milk are the commonest culprits, but these have usually faded by the age of 13 years. Peanuts and tree nut allergies are becoming increasingly common. Shellfish and white fish (cod) allergies are less common but usually easy to identify.

9.10 Why do some people react to fresh food but not to the same food when it is cooked?

This is frequently encountered, and most often reflects a cross-reaction between proteins in birch pollen and similar proteins in fruit from trees of the *Rosacea* family (*Table 9.1*). This family includes apples, pears, apricots,

TABLE 9.1 Cross-reactivity between foods and other allergens

Allergen	Cross-reacting foods
Birch (Bet v1)	Apple, pear, peach, nectarine, plum, cherry, apricot, celery
Birch (Bet v2 — profilin)	Carrot, celery, potato, buckwheat
Tropomyosin (in house dust mite — Der p10)	Shrimp, snails, other shellfish
Latex (Hev b5)	Kiwifruit
Latex (heveins)	Avocado, banana, chestnut

peaches, cherries, plums, greengages and almonds. The fruit proteins are altered by cooking and so it is safe to eat jam, cooked fruit and most fruit juices. Similar cross-reactions can occur with carrot, potato, celery and pepper, which cross-react with different pollen species. People with latex allergy commonly react to banana, chestnut, papaya and mango, although the fruit proteins here may be more resistant to cooking.

9.11 Is coeliac disease a food allergy?

Strictly speaking it is an allergic response to food and so it should be classified as a food allergy. However, the mechanisms involved are quite different from most of the other forms of food allergy. Coeliac disease (also known as gluten-sensitive enteropathy) is caused by an immunological response to gluten proteins in wheat. The gluten is recognized by T cells which cause damage to the lining of the small bowel. The damaged small bowel is unable to absorb nutrients properly and the patient becomes malnourished.

9.12 What is dermatitis herpetiformis and how does it relate to coeliac disease?

Dermatitis herpetiformis is an itchy rash typically affecting the upper arms, but may be anywhere on body. Immunologically and clinically, the condition is linked to gluten sensitivity and responds to a gluten-free diet.

DIAGNOSIS

9.13 What should be done for the patient who thinks they have a food allergy?

First and most important, a full history of the reactions that the patient thinks may be related to food should be taken. Without arguing with the patient, try to separate out what happened from what the patient believes to be the cause. The time between the ingestion of the suspect food and the episode is a critical factor in assessing the relevance of the food. Most immediate-type reactions will happen within 1 h of ingestion, rarely up to 2 h after ingestion, but it is most unlikely that something eaten 6–12 h earlier will be responsible for new symptoms. Diagnostic tests should be used to help validate the history and should never be the sole basis of a diagnosis of food allergy.

9.14 What if a patient appears to react to numerous foods?

As always in allergy, it is most important to obtain a clear history of the nature of the reactions, and their relationship to the suspect foods. It is also worth checking carefully whether the patient has been able to eat any of the suspected trigger foods without problems since the onset of their symptoms. In some cases, the allergic reactions may appear to be independent of food; in other cases there may be a more convincing relationship.

9.15 Which tests are useful in suspected food allergy?

There is no single test for identifying and diagnosing food allergy. Skin prick tests allow a large number of allergens to be tested in the clinic, with immediate results and low overall cost. Blood tests (usually called RASTs (radioallergosorbent tests) but which often employ more advanced technology) are useful when suitable skin test extracts are not available or when skin tests are technically unsatisfactory. Both tests will identify food-specific IgE responses but neither will help validate a diagnosis of food intolerance (which is based on the history alone). Skin tests are slightly more sensitive (i.e. they will detect lower levels of antibody).

9.16 How reliable are food allergy skin tests?

The predictive value of food allergy skin tests varies from one food to another. For some allergens, such as cod and other white fishes, almost everyone with a positive skin test has symptoms, and almost everyone with symptoms has a positive skin test. For peanuts, everyone with significant symptoms will have a positive skin test, but so will a significant number of people who have no symptoms on exposure. With wheat, huge numbers of symptom-free people will have positive skin tests (including most people with grass pollen hay fever). Most of these will be asymptomatic if they eat wheat. Thus a positive result demonstrates sensitivity but not necessarily allergy. However, a negative result can be taken as evidence that the patient is not sensitized.

9.17 How does one diagnose adverse food reactions?

The history is the key to assessing food reactions. If allergy is truly responsible, then in most cases the relationship between the food and the symptoms will be clear. For classical food allergy, supportive evidence should be obtained by skin or blood tests for specific IgE, and there is no need to proceed to oral challenge tests. The suspect food should be removed from the diet and the patient should be followed up to see if the problem recurs.

If the history is doubtful and investigations prove negative, the patient can be reassured and allowed to revert to a normal diet. When the initial event was mild, rechallenge can be done at home. However, when the patient had a significant episode, but investigation suggests it is not caused by food allergy, it may be best to rechallenge under medical supervision.

This allows the patient to have confidence in eating the suspect food, and also means that if the investigations have provided false reassurance, you will find out in clinic rather than in the pub!

9.18 How is an elimination diet conducted?

Before starting on an elimination diet, it is important to reach a view on whether the symptoms presented by the patient are likely to have any allergic basis. Patients should be discouraged from starting on broad elimination diets without first seeking medical advice. Input from a dietitian is always helpful, both to ensure that the suspect foods really are excluded and to ensure adequate calorie and vitamin intake. The choice of foods to exclude may be based on allergy skin tests, i.e. the diet serves to validate the skin tests. Alternatively, in conditions such as irritable bowel syndrome, the diet may be more empirical. It is known that many patients with IBS have difficulty digesting wheat and dairy products, so it can be worth eliminating these for a while (6–8 weeks) to see if there is any improvement. When an improvement is found, it can be worth rechallenging the patient to make sure that the dietary restriction is truly justified (see below).

9.19 How is a food challenge conducted?

At its simplest, a patient may be asked to eat a small quantity of the suspect food in its natural form. This is an open challenge, and would be appropriate if the original symptoms were clear and no evidence had been found of allergy on skin or blood tests. The main purpose of the open challenge is thus to reassure the patient that it is safe to eat a suspect food. In other settings, where the symptoms are less easy to define, and where the link between the food and the symptoms is uncertain, it is preferable to perform challenges in a blinded manner. The gold standard is a double-blind placebo-controlled procedure, in which the patient receives the food in a disguised form on one day, and then has a dummy challenge on another day. Neither the patient nor the doctor should know which day is which, until the effects of each challenge have been recorded. Double-blind placebo-controlled challenges are very time-consuming to perform; they are useful for research purposes, but in clinical practice they should be reserved for those cases where it is really essential to know whether food allergy is present.

9.20 Are VEGA tests useful for diagnosing food allergies?

No. Electrical tests of skin are widely used by nutritionists and other practitioners of complementary medicine, but independent evaluations have not been able to validate the basis of the test. See Chapter 12 for full explanation.

9.21   How can one diagnose coeliac disease and dermatitis herpetiformis?

In the past, the diagnosis was confirmed by finding histological abnormalities on jejunal biopsy that recover when the patient goes onto a gluten-free diet. An accurate diagnosis is essential since the therapy is lifelong and there are other abnormalities of the small bowel which can look like gluten-sensitive enteropathy (GSE). Gluten-free diets should not be prescribed until the intestinal biopsy has been performed as the histological appearances will revert towards normal soon after starting the diet, and it may be difficult to confirm the diagnosis. Ideally, the biopsy should be repeated once the patient is established on the diet and again after rechallenging with gluten. However, most physicians are reluctant to subject patients with obvious GSE to three biopsies.

Nowadays, there are useful screening tests for antibodies directed against wheat proteins. Anti-gliadin and anti-endomysial antibodies are positive in virtually all patients who have GSE, and these tests are therefore useful in excluding patients who do not have GSE and thereby can be spared the need for jejunal biopsy. For patients in whom a positive anti-wheat antibody titre is found, it is still appropriate to proceed to jejunal biopsy, as there are false-positive antibody results (i.e. people who have positive antibody titres but do not have coeliac disease on jejunal biopsy).

9.22   Can patients be allergic to alcohol?

Allergy-like symptoms after ingesting alcohol are relatively frequent, but these do not involve true allergy to the alcohol itself. It is important to take a careful history, including the precise circumstances when the reaction occurs, and whether it occurs with all or just some forms of alcohol.

Some patients are sensitive to the histamine and other fermentation products in wine; others react to the sulphites that are used to keep white wine clear (otherwise it oxidizes and goes a cloudy brown colour). Sulphametabisulphite is used in the cleaning of equipment in home brewing and wine making, and high levels may be found in the resulting brew. Some additives, such as tartrazine and sodium benzoate, can trigger urticaria and asthma.

Some patients are allergic to yeast (more often a problem with beer and wine than with spirits). Allergy to the fruit (grapes, apples, juniper berries, coconuts, oranges), hops or grains from which the drink is made could theoretically cause a true allergy. Alcohol dilates small blood vessels and can thus exacerbate underlying conditions such as migraine, rhinitis, urticaria or asthma by dilating the blood vessels. Finally, some people, especially those from oriental races, do not have the alcohol dehydrogenase enzyme which allows most westerners to degrade alcohol. People who are deficient in alcohol dehydrogenase will flush with relatively small amounts of any form of alcohol, and this may be mistaken for an allergy.

Alcohol also increases the permeability of the gut, facilitating the absorption of food molecules. This may explain the phenomenon of the patient with a mild food sensitivity who only reacts to food when it is combined with alcohol.

9.23 Can food cause contact dermatitis?

Some foods can cause local irritation, because they contain either irritants (e.g. pimento, paprika, etc.) or histamine (e.g. salami). Most often this will show up as local irritation around the mouth. Allergy to egg and cow's milk can contribute to atopic eczema, but this is not driven by direct contact of the food with the skin and shows up in the usual places for atopic eczema.

MANAGEMENT

9.24 How should children with egg or milk allergy be managed?

Children who are milk-allergic should avoid all forms of milk or milk products, including butter, yoghurts, cream, cheese, etc. They will require calcium and vitamin D supplementation. Children on an egg-restricted diet will often have to eliminate a huge range of food from their diet. Most cakes, biscuits, chocolates, soups, sauces, custards, ice-creams, pancakes, sweet breads, pastries and batters contain egg or egg-derived substrates. The help of a dietitian is essential to help maintain a varied and nutritionally adequate diet. Assistance in shopping for egg-free products can be obtained from supermarkets who offer lists of prepared and packaged foods which are egg-free.

9.25 Is goat or sheep milk an acceptable substitute in cow's milk allergy?

In children with true cow's milk allergy, these milks should all be avoided, as the antibodies are directed against proteins in cow's milk which are very similar to those in sheep and goat milk. However, in people with cow's milk intolerance, it is common to find that the problem is because of the fat composition of the milk, and so they will notice improvements with alternative ruminant milks. Failure to draw this distinction accurately has led to some controversy and argument in the lay and medical press.

9.26 Should children with cow's milk allergy be rechallenged and, if so, when?

Cautious reintroduction of prohibited foods should be attempted after 6–12 months. The natural history of food allergy in many children is gradual improvement of symptoms even though the skin tests remain positive. Many children eventually develop tolerance to milk and eggs but rarely to fish or to nuts, although there is data suggesting that 20% of children with peanut allergy will have lost this by the time they are 18-years-old.

9.27 Which drugs are useful in food allergy?

Drug treatment is only indicated in food allergy when symptoms persist despite attempts at an elimination diet. This may occur if diagnosis is incomplete, exposure is unavoidable or the patient is poorly compliant. None of the drugs available are perfect: preventative drugs for food allergy include oral sodium cromoglycate (Nalcrom) and ketotifen (Zaditen). Symptom-relieving medication should be chosen on the basis of the symptoms experienced (bronchodilators and inhaled steroids for asthma, topical steroids for eczema, antihistamines for food-induced urticaria, and adrenaline for life-threatening anaphylaxis).

9.28 Where can patients with coeliac disease get advice on what is safe to eat?

The Coeliac Society publishes an annual list of manufactured products that are gluten-free (see Appendix).

9.29 Are wheat-free and gluten-free diets synonymous?

No. Gluten is a mixture of proteins found in wheat and in smaller amounts in some other cereals. Consequently, foods that are only gluten-free are not suitable for a wheat-free diet unless the product also states wheat-free, indicating that no wheat has been used at all.

The presence or possible presence of wheat in a food is indicated by the following words: bran, wheat bran, cereal filler, cereal binder, cereal protein, couscous, farina, flour, whole-wheat flour, wheat flour, wheat starch, rusk, semolina, starch, modified starch, hydrolysed starch, food starch, edible starch, vegetable starch, vegetable gum, vegetable protein, wheatgerm, wheat (durum, spelt, kamut).

9.30 What are the alternatives to wheat?

The alternative cereals include rye, oats, barley, corn and rice. In addition, there are more unusual flours such as arrowroot, amaranth, bean, buckwheat, lentil, millet, pea, potato, quinoa and soya.

9.31 If a patient is allergic to fish should they avoid shellfish too?

Fish and shellfish are two distinct categories of food, and the immunological responses are directed against distinct proteins. Other types of fish such as tuna, salmon and trout also have their own antigens. Thus, unless the patient gives a history of problems they need only avoid the class of food to which they are allergic. Ideally, individuals with fish allergy should also be tested for shellfish allergy so that they are aware of their allergic status with respect to shellfish.

However, there is potential for cross-contamination in the preparation of these foods. Fish and shellfish may be handled together at the fish market, displayed together in a restaurant or shop and prepared together in the kitchen. For these reasons, many individuals with fish allergy may choose to avoid all seafood.

Similar considerations apply to peanuts and tree nuts.

9.32 Where else might fish be hidden?

A person allergic to fish needs to be vigilant in a number of settings. Anchovies are frequently used in salad sauces and pizza toppings. Caesar salad dressing, Worcestershire sauce and barbecue sauces frequently contain anchovies.

Crab sticks, those bright pink imitation sticks of crab, are typically made from white fish such as pollack. Various Asian dishes use fish sauce as a flavouring base.

9.33 What should I advise my patients with oral allergy syndrome?

In most patients this is a nuisance rather than a serious problem. Patients who are aware of the nature of their mouth symptoms may prefer to avoid the offending foods; others may enjoy the food and be prepared to put up with the mouth symptoms. Those who wish to reduce the symptoms will either have to avoid the fresh fruits or take an antihistamine before eating an apple, etc. At present it does not seem that desensitizing people to tree pollen has any effect on oral allergy syndrome.

PROGNOSIS

9.34 Do people grow out of their food allergies?

Yes, but it varies according to the foodstuff involved and the age of the patient. Children with cow's milk and egg allergy will usually lose this by the time they are 10 years of age. Of children with proven peanut allergy, 20% will lose this by 18 years. Most adults with allergy to shellfish, cod or nuts will continue to have this for the rest of their lives.

9.35 What advice should be given to a mother about breast feeding further children when one child has a documented food allergy?

In general, atopic mothers and mothers of atopic children should not wean their children early. Breast feeding for 6 months should allow the baby's immune system to mature and thereby become less likely to develop allergies to new foods. If breast feeding is not sufficient, hydrolysed soy-based infant formulas are probably the best option, although the evidence to support this is somewhat soft. Avoiding smoking while pregnant and during the first year of baby's life is still the most effective way of reducing the likelihood of the baby developing allergies.

THE FUTURE

9.36 Is it likely that desensitization will soon be available for food allergies or oral allergy syndrome?

Several strategies are being used to try to suppress peanut allergy. These include prototype vaccines and sophisticated efforts to 'silence' the relevant genes in peanuts. These are still at early stages and it is not clear when these might become widely available.

For the oral allergy syndrome, people have tried using tree pollen vaccine. This deals with the birch pollen allergy but has not proved effective against the cross-reactions that cause the symptoms of the oral allergy syndrome, so is not currently recommended.

9.37 Is the advice on managing food allergy likely to change?

Advice should change as the knowledge base changes. Likely trends would be in the areas of prevention, where there is current controversy about whether the gut and the immune system can be protected by early introduction of boiled peanuts, or more general approaches based on the hygiene hypothesis (altering the gut bacterial flora to bias the system towards tolerance rather than allergy) (*Question 1.41*).

9.38 Could genetically modified foods cause allergy in the future?

Genetic modification is undertaken for two distinct reasons: to improve crop yield and to give the plant a defensive advantage against parasites and weather. Simple improvements in crop yield will just give increased amounts per acre of the standard crop proteins. This form of genetic modification is no different to the series of breeding improvements made in wheat cultivation over past millennia. More complex modifications may introduce foreign proteins which are nutritionally advantageous, but could present unintended allergic hazards, e.g. putting a nut protein into soya to increase and alter the protein content of the grain. Proteins introduced into plants to protect them against insect parasites may be allergenic in their own right, so some caution is required. Proteins introduced to alter weather-resistance might involve quite major cross-species exchanges, e.g. arctic fish genes put into tomatoes to reduce their sensitivity to frost, with the potential for fish-allergic people to react to GM tomatoes!

PATIENT QUESTIONS

9.39 Do nut-allergic patients have to avoid nut oil?

The allergy is to proteins in the peanuts or tree nuts. Conventional oils should not contain any protein and, indeed, there have been studies showing that patients with extreme levels of nut allergy do not react to ingestion of 50 ml of peanut oil. However, some gourmet oils (used for making salads and dressings) are deliberately produced with some nut protein ground in for flavour. These oils are theoretically less safe but have not been shown to be dangerous. In practical terms, it is not necessary to check which oil is being used at the chip-shop or for frying crisps.

9.40 Are all forms of peanut equally dangerous to nut-allergic patients?

There is good evidence that dry roasting has less effect on the peanut proteins than boiling them. So the techniques used in the West for making peanut snacks and peanut butter preserve the allergens more than oriental styles of cooking.

9.41 What is the current advice regarding egg allergy and MMR?

Egg allergy is not a contraindication to MMR (measles, mumps, rubella) vaccination. The current advice is that, for those children who have experienced a very severe allergic reaction to egg, the vaccination should be given in a hospital setting, where the vaccine can be given by someone trained and equipped to deal with the very small chance of a reaction. Where the allergy is mild the vaccination may be given in the community. For children with allergy to antibiotics or latex it is also advisable for the vaccination to be given in a hospital setting.

Patients should be advised not to be put off this vaccination, or other vaccinations offered to small children if their child has an egg allergy. None of the other vaccines contain egg protein and, in the case of MMR vaccine, even taking into account an egg allergy, the risks of the disease themselves are much greater than those of the vaccination.

9.42 What is Chinese Restaurant Syndrome?

This is an example of a food intolerance in that it is thought to be caused by monosodium glutamate (MSG). MSG is a flavour-enhancer that is added to many foodstuffs (*Box 9.1*). Its flavour-enhancing properties are dependent on the depolarizing or excitatory action it has on sensory taste receptors. The amino acid glutamic acid is an important component of all proteins, and in this form it is well tolerated in the diet. Reactions are thought to occur when it is ingested as glutamate. Although glutamate is present naturally in mushrooms and tomatoes, it has not been noted to cause problems when it occurs naturally. It has also been difficult to reproduce Chinese Restaurant Syndrome in the laboratory.

BOX 9.1 Foods containing monosodium glutamate (MSG)

Chinese food (one bowl of Wonton soup can contain as much as
2.5 g MSG)
Highly seasoned prepared and restaurant food
Proprietary flavour-enhancers (e.g. Aromat)
Cheeses (100 g Camembert may contain 1 g MSG)
Tomatoes
Mushrooms
Instant soups and gravies

The typical symptoms of Chinese Restaurant Syndrome are headache, a
burning sensation along the back of the neck, chest tightness or pain, nausea,
sweating and a sensation of facial or intraorbital pressure. Pins or needles or
tingling may be experienced in the limbs, face and head. In adults, a
threshold dose of 1.5–3.0 g is required before symptoms occur, and reactions
are more likely to occur if MSG is eaten on an empty stomach. It has been
estimated that as many as 30% of the adult population may be affected, with
females more susceptible than males.

9.43 Do children suffer from Chinese Restaurant Syndrome?

It is not entirely clear, but it is commonly thought that young children may
experience shivering or shudder attacks and older children migraine after
consuming MSG.

9.44 Are there any other problems associated with MSG ingestion?

Yes. MSG can provoke asthma in those who already have the condition. Two
patterns are recognized: an early response occurring 1–2 h after ingestion or a
late reaction occurring after 10–14 h. MSG can also trigger cutaneous lesions
such as urticaria.

9.45 How useful are lists of safe food?

These are enormously helpful when planning a menu or shopping list.
However, it is not uncommon for manufacturers to change the ingredients
of a product and they may do so without warning. Additionally, ingredients
can vary between the different sizes of the same product, e.g. regular size and
mini size chocolate bars. For these reasons, lists of safe foods are helpful but
are no substitute for reading the labels.

9.46 How big a problem is cross-contamination?

This is really an issue only for those with extreme levels of sensitivity.
Production lines used for one form of confectionery will be cleaned before a
new line is produced, but small traces or chips of nut may remain in the
machine and contaminate the next product. Food may be contaminated in
preparation (e.g. frying different foods in the same deep fryers). Individual

items may become contaminated at the retail level (e.g. in handling bakery goods). Finally, food may become contaminated by spillage or inadvertent transfer (e.g. nuts falling into tubs of ice-cream, pick and mix sweet displays).

9.47 How can I get help with shopping?

Shopping for people with food intolerance can be time-consuming and frustrating. Specialized 'Free from' lists are available for milk-free, egg-free, wheat-free, gluten-free, soya-free, nut- and peanut-free, preservative-free, vegan and vegetarian diets. These are usually available within larger supermarkets or from their head offices. Major manufacturers such as Walkers, Heinz and Findus also produce similar lists relating to their own produce.

Dietitians have access to lists produced by the food intolerance databank. The advantage of these is they are available for multiple dietary exclusions (e.g. free from wheat, eggs and milk) as well as single exclusions (e.g. soya). The lists are not exhaustive as they contain only information from those supermarkets and manufacturers who wish to be included.

Local health food shops are the best source of special diet products and are often willing to order from catalogues the products not on their shelves. The larger supermarkets are increasingly stocking special diet products, e.g. gluten-free pasta, soya ice-cream and yoghurt, dairy-free cheeses. Unlike the health food shops, these products are often widely dispersed within the supermarket, and may sometimes be found in the organic section as well.

Manufacturers of special products such as dairy-free margarine, egg replacer, etc. often produce recipe leaflets. Some companies (particularly the gluten-free and wheat-free product companies) produce videos and demonstrations. The Coeliac Society has details of these.

The internet provides an excellent source of information, recipes and shopping opportunities. Typing in 'special diet cookery' or 'special diet recipes' will link you with many informative and helpful sites. www.allergyfreedirect.co.uk sell special dietary products by mail order and also offer cakes and biscuits made to your own specifications and recipes.

Special diet cookbooks are available from health food shops, book shops, internet book retailers and from allergy associations such as Allergy UK and Action Against Allergy.

9.48 Is food labelling really helpful?

Supermarkets and food manufacturers are tending to supply more informative labelling about allergens on their products, e.g. suitable for a milk-free diet, egg-free, contains gluten.

However, the phrase 'may contain traces of nut' is causing much controversy. Its almost universal use on confectionery, bakery and cereals is unhelpful and is seen as a 'cop out' by the food industry.

For vegetable oils also there is no requirement to be specific. Vegetable oil could refer to corn oil or groundnut oil. Therefore individuals wanting to avoid peanut oil have currently to avoid all foodstuffs labelled vegetable.

Patient advice agencies and consumer pressure groups are currently working with industry to try to reach a more useful labelling policy.

Some current anomalies in food labelling cause difficulty. Present EU regulation about food labelling requires products to display the components of constituent parts only if they constitute more than 25% of the final product. So, for example, pizza with a pepperoni and Milanese sauce topping would only need to list these and would not have to detail the constituent ingredients if the pepperoni or sauce made up less than 25% of the total weight.

9.49 Should I be worried about flying if I have a food allergy?

Anyone with a serious food allergy should inform their airline, *at the time of booking the flight*, so that they can be sure of receiving an appropriate allergen-free meal. Because of the air circulation in aircraft it is possible for small particles containing peanut allergens to be circulated if packets of peanuts are handed out to passengers with cocktails. Some airlines (including British Airways) have stopped serving peanuts to protect their allergic passengers; other airlines have decided that the risk is theoretical and small and does not require action.

9.50 Should nut-allergic people avoid all nuts?

Some patients react only to one type of nut (this is more often observed with brazil nuts or cashews than with peanuts). Others react to most tree nuts (walnut, brazil, cashew, hazel, almond, macadamia, pistachio etc.) but not to peanuts, while others may react to all types of nut including peanuts. Skin tests are useful here: if the history and tests are negative, then it is safe to eat the nuts. Some people who are clinically allergic to peanuts have positive skin tests to one or more tree nuts but no history of symptoms. This indicates that they do have antibodies against the tree nuts, but it is usually safe to continue to eat those nuts to which they have no symptoms. However, when dining out or travelling abroad, it is probably best to avoid all nuts.

Occupational allergies

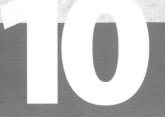

PQ PATIENT QUESTIONS

INTRODUCTION

10.1 How common are occupational allergies?

Occupational asthma is now the commonest form of occupational lung disease and is thought to account for 5–10% of all adult-onset asthma. Occupational skin disease is common in certain occupations, but can be minimized by proper occupational hygiene. Occupational rhinitis is also well recognized, generally in the same groups that suffer from occupational asthma, although the causes and prevalence are less well defined than for asthma.

10.2 In which occupations are patients most at risk of developing an allergy? (See *Table 10.1*)

Occupational asthma is particularly common among people working with animals, e.g. vets, pet-shop workers, laboratory animal handlers, etc. Both small and large animals are problematic, with horses, cats and rodents being the most potent sensitizers. Bakers and others handling flour may become sensitized both to the flour and to enzymes such as amylase that are added to flour before baking. Paint sprayers, especially those working in car body

TABLE 10.1 Allergens and jobs frequently associated with occupational asthma	
Allergens	**Occupation**
Laboratory animals	Research workers
Drugs, e.g. antibiotics, psyllium	Pharmaceutical industry
Plants	Healthcare (latex)
	Brewery (hops)
	Tea industry
	Cabinet makers
Birds	Bird fanciers
	Poultry farmers
Enzymes	Bakers (amylase)
	Detergent manufacturer
Flour	Bakers
Fish/shellfish/crab	Fish processing plants
Insects	Grain workers (mites)
	Florists
	Greenhouse workers
Colophony	Soldering, electronics assembly
Acid anhydrides	Electronics industry
Isocyanates	Painters, body shops
	Plastic manufacturer

shops, are at high risk of sensitization to isocyanates. Hairdressers and barbers can become sensitized to dyes, bleaches and aerosols, which cause both asthma and eczema. Woodworkers and people working in the plastics and electronics industries are also at risk. Healthcare workers are at increased risk of allergy to latex (rubber), which can cause both contact eczema and occupational asthma. Any job that involves the use of solvents may make asthma worse, and those with dust mite allergies will find difficulty in jobs that involve cleaning (chamber maids, domestic cleaners, etc.).

10.3 Are there jobs that people with allergies cannot do?

People with asthma are generally excluded from baking and paint spraying because of the risk that they may develop occupational sensitization. Asthmatics are also unlikely to be employed in the armed forces or police service because the high level of fitness required increases the rate of drop-out from training among asthmatic recruits. People with hand eczema should avoid jobs that involve frequent washing or wet hands (e.g. healthcare, bar work, hairdressing, etc.). Latex allergy is a major problem in healthcare workers, who are usually screened for contact allergy before starting work. Redeployment is the preferred option for trained staff, but some branches of healthcare will be impractical for those found to have latex allergy.

DIAGNOSIS

10.4 If a patient presents with a concern about occupational exposure how should this be approached?

The most important thing to do is obtain a clear history of the patient's problem and their reasons for thinking that it may be work-related. Careful reference to old notes may help to clarify whether the presentation is really a new problem, or an exacerbation of a pre-existing condition. If the history is suggestive, the patient will probably need to be referred for specialist investigation. Removing someone from the workplace usually results in significant financial loss for the worker, who should not be advised without establishing a clear diagnosis and a basis for compensation through the courts or social security.

10.5 When should occupational asthma be considered?

The possibility of occupational causes should be considered in all patients with adult-onset asthma even if the patient does not suspect a link. Conversely, anyone who becomes breathless while working in an industry that is known to cause occupational asthma may present to the GP claiming they have developed occupational asthma. Some of these will have conditions other than asthma, but their concerns need to be taken seriously, especially if they are threatened with losing their job.

10.6 When should occupational eczema be considered?

Anyone presenting with contact eczema should be asked about their work, and whether there is any relationship between their eczema and work. Those in high-risk occupations may already be aware of the possibility. Those working with chemicals should be asked to obtain copies of data sheets relating to the processes and raw materials to which they are being exposed.

10.7 Is asthma in the workplace always occupational asthma?

Some patients will have pre-existing asthma that has been made worse by dusty conditions in the workplace. In some of these cases the underlying diagnosis may have gone unrecognized, but in retrospect the patient has had childhood symptoms compatible with asthma. Others will have clear cut new onset asthma in the workplace, with no pre-existing symptoms, and a third group will have a combination (i.e. mild pre-existing asthma, with subsequent sensitization to an occupational allergen which is making the asthma worse). This group is the most difficult in which to achieve an agreed diagnosis. Finally, there is a group of patients with asthma symptoms that develop after massive exposure to irritant vapours, smoke, etc. These are generally classified as industrial injuries rather than true occupational asthma.

10.8 Is occupational asthma always allergic in origin?

True occupational asthma involves immune recognition of one or more agents encountered in the workplace, and is thus always allergic in origin. Patients with irritant-induced asthma (sometimes called reactive airways dysfunction syndrome or RADS) will have asthmatic symptoms, but this group does not have allergic sensitization.

MANAGEMENT

10.9 Are there occasions when changing jobs will not relieve the symptoms?

Unfortunately, a proportion of patients with occupational asthma, perhaps as much as one-third, will not improve despite complete avoidance of the agent that caused their problem. The likelihood of persistent symptoms is increased the longer the patient continues to work after developing symptoms, and is also increased in those with the heaviest exposure to the inciting agent.

10.10 What advice should be given to dermatitis sufferers at work?

Minimize exposure to irritant and sensitizing chemicals, wear protective equipment that is provided and insist on good quality protective equipment if what is provided is not adequate. Treat any hand eczema with emollients and prescribed medication.

10.11 Is allergic occupational disease notifiable?

Not in the sense that infectious diseases are notifiable. However, sufferers should inform their occupational health service and their union representative (if applicable). The Health and Safety Executive may also be asked to investigate, either by management or the employee.

10.12 Is it possible to receive compensation for occupational asthma?

Yes, it is relatively simple to obtain state compensation for occupational asthma, but the amount received is quite low, and rarely compensates for the loss of earnings if the patient has to leave their job. Consequently, many employees will need to make a claim against their employers. To obtain compensation in the courts, it is necessary to show injury, and also that the employer was negligent in their duty of care to the employees. The standard of proof for compensation in the courts is based on the balance of probabilities, but this is somewhat higher than that required by the state compensation scheme, so some patients are able to get state compensation, but have little chance of winning a court case.

10.13 What career advice should be offered to a 14-year-old with a strong history of atopy?

It is probably best to avoid occupations in which there is a high rate of occupational allergy (see above). If the young person is convinced about a particular career that carries such a risk, they need to go in with their eyes open, and they should also be advised to take extra care to minimize their exposure (both by inhalation and skin contact).

PROGNOSIS

10.14 Will occupational asthma disappear if the patient stops work?

The patient does not necessarily have to stop work to avoid the inciting agent and, provided exposure can be avoided, redeployment in the same workplace is usually the best option. In true occupational asthma, about one-third of patients will lose their asthma altogether if they are able to avoid the agent to which they have become sensitized. Another third will improve noticeably, but will continue to experience some asthmatic symptoms, but about 30% will not improve, even though they manage to avoid the inciting agent completely. This does not mean that their asthma is non-occupational; rather it implies that the occupational agent was responsible for starting the asthma process, and this has now become independent of the original trigger.

10.15 Is there anything that can be done to accelerate the process of resolution?

Apart from removing the patient from exposure, there is nothing that has been proven to work. It is an article of faith that patients with occupational asthma should be treated aggressively with inhaled steroids and other anti-asthma medication, but no controlled studies have been reported as showing any increase in the rate of resolution or the proportion of patients whose asthma resolves.

THE FUTURE

10.16 Will the incidence of occupational asthma continue to increase?

The key to reducing the burden of occupational asthma is industrial hygiene. Early indications are that the number of new cases is reaching a plateau, although new causes of occupational asthma continue to be recognized each year. In the next 25 years, we can expect to see an increasing number of cases of malignant mesothelioma (caused by asbestos), which will soon displace occupational asthma as the commonest occupational lung disease.

10.17 Can we expect any developments in the care of occupational asthma?

Occupational asthma is one of the forms of asthma in which the condition truly disappears. It is also the only setting in which one sees reversal of the subepithelial basement membrane thickening that is typically found in asthma. This thickening has been associated with the production of the growth factor TNFα, and it has therefore been suggested that targeting TNFα or other relevant cytokines might accelerate the process of resolution of occupational asthma.

PQ   PATIENT QUESTIONS

10.18 What are the employer's responsibilities to a person who has developed an allergy in the workplace?

The employer has a duty of care to his employees. This includes a duty to avoid exposing workers to unnecessary or known hazards. Employers are obliged to provide workers with material safety data sheets on all chemicals being used in the workplace, including details of their potential to cause occupational sensitization, eczema and asthma. Larger employers also have obligations to provide appropriate occupational health services, which should advise the employer on hazards reported to them, as well as taking care of the workers.

10.19 Does smoking increase the risk of occupational asthma?

For some allergens but not for others. People working with acid anhydrides are more likely to become sensitized if they are atopic (with sensitivity to grass pollen, house dust mite, etc.), but they are unlikely to develop symptomatic occupational asthma unless they also smoke. The mechanism of this interaction is not known, but cigarette smoke is known to promote the production of IgE antibody. Alternatively, smoke may damage the integrity of the airway and allow chemicals to gain access to the underlying immune system.

Allergy in children

INTRODUCTION

11.1 Why do so many children have allergies nowadays? Is it genetic?

'Allergy is the price paid by the children of the wealthy middle classes for their current relative freedom from the diseases which have afflicted humanity throughout its evolution'. This view, expressed in the mid-1970s, encapsulates much current thinking on the causes of the recent rise in allergic disease.

> Of one thing we can be sure, while allergy has a strong genetic component, being seen in families and passed from one generation to the next, the causes of the recent rise in allergies cannot be blamed on genetics. Over long periods of time the range and variety of genetic differences in a population will change, but this cannot happen in a single generation, unless there is an extreme selection pressure, such as a plague which wipes out a large proportion of the population. Something like this may have happened in Europe during the Black Death, when perhaps as much as one-third of the population of Europe died. Those that survived may well have been less susceptible to the effects of the plague, and hence their genes would have been more likely to pass to the next generation. However, in modern times, the genetic pool of each generation is derived from the previous generation with very little change.

11.2 Is the increase in allergic children real or just diagnostic fashion?

In the 1970s and 1980s there was a dramatic increase in the number of children seeing their GPs for asthma (*Fig. 11.1*). On its own, this does not prove that there is more asthma, as it could be caused simply by people being quicker to consult their doctor. However, epidemiological studies using the same questions several years apart have shown a true increase in the number of children with asthma. The best UK data is from Aberdeen and suggests that between 1964 and 1989 there was a 2.5-fold increase in the rate of asthma in children aged 7–10 years, and a threefold increase in hay fever and eczema. We can assume that the children who developed asthma and allergies in 1964 would also have done so if they had been born 25 years later, but the excess must consist of children who would not have developed allergic disorders if they had been born in the 1950s. Looking further back, there is tantalizing evidence that asthma was rare in the 19th century: Charles Bostock wrote a treatise on hay fever in the 1860s, and took 5 years to find seven cases of hay fever, including his own.

Taken together, this epidemiological evidence suggests that there was a cohort of children who developed asthma and allergies in the 1930s–1950s.

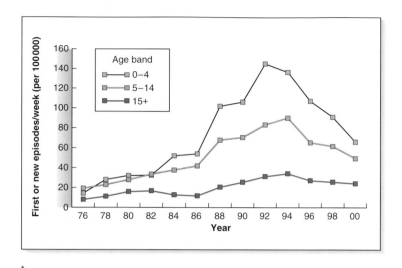

▲

Fig 11.1 Consultation rates for asthma in England and Wales 1976-2000. Adapted from the Lung Information Agency.

This group must have had a genetic tendency to do so and this was exposed by changes in the environment that were operating in the UK before 1960. The more recent rise represents a separate cohort who were resistant to the environmental changes at work before 1960, but whose genetic tendency was exposed by environmental changes that occurred around or shortly after 1960.

11.3   If it isn't genetic, is it to do with modern lifestyles?

Some clues can be obtained from observations that allergic disease was and remains more prevalent among the better off. However, this could be caused by a wide range of factors, including smaller family size, better housing conditions, boarding schools, etc. More persuasive evidence that the rise is linked to lifestyle comes from Germany, where detailed studies have been made of children in the former East and West Germany. For all practical purposes the populations of East and West Germany are genetically identical, although there are some regional ethnic variations that arose from the forced repatriation of Germans from Eastern Europe after 1945. At the time of reunification in 1989/1990, the rates of allergic sensitization and asthma were markedly higher in West than in East Germany. This was thought at the time to be related to differences in air pollution, and several epidemiological studies were started. It has been shown that, among those born before 1960, the rates of allergic sensitization and disease are identical in the East and West. In those born after 1960 a gradually increasing gap appears, with those born in the West more and more likely to develop allergies. Conversely, the rates of allergies in the East remain constant across this 29-year period. By the time that those born in 1989 are considered, the difference is 2.5-fold, very similar to the differences observed in the UK between those aged 7 and 10 years in 1964 and 1989 in the Aberdeen data discussed above. The implications are: (1) allergy is being driven by something associated with the post-1960 German economic miracle; and (2) that the critical period is at, or around the time of, birth, so those born in 1960 retained the risk of allergic disease with which they were born, despite living in the increasingly affluent West.

Several possible factors have been suggested, and it may well be that this rise is driven by a combination of factors, or by different combinations in different individuals. The front runners follow:

- Housing-related: many different changes that have made our homes more comfortable for house dust mites.
- Dietary: changes in food technology associated with supermarkets, etc.
- Gut microflora: we know that the infant gut is colonized with bacteria soon after birth, and the composition of the gut flora directly reflects the mother's own gut flora. Intestinal bacteria are the single most important factor in shaping the newborn immune system, and are responsible for:
  — switching the immune system over to a defensive configuration (as opposed to the passive configuration that is desirable in the womb)
  — shaping the T cell repertoire (the range of things that T lymphocytes can recognize as foreign)
  — forming the lymphoid organs and nodes (animals that are raised in a sterile environment do not form recognizable lymph nodes).

11.4   What is the Allergic March?

It is well recognized that some children become sensitized during infancy, and then go on to develop eczema in early childhood, followed by allergic asthma or rhinitis in later childhood. While it is clear that these conditions share risk factors, it is less certain whether each one leads to the other. The Allergic March is a hypothesis that these are stages that are linked and each leads to the next. Hence it might be possible to interrupt the sequence by early identification of at-risk individuals and appropriate intervention(s). Research is currently assessing the true nature of the rates of progression from one stage to the next, as well as some preliminary studies investigating whether interventions can prevent progression.

DIAGNOSIS

11.5 Which tests can be done in children of different ages?

Skin prick tests can be performed in very young children, but their diagnostic value is limited before 3 years of age. Blood tests are less appropriate than skin tests. Simple lung function can be performed in children as young as 3 years, but their value increases as the child grows (*see Questions 2.9 and 11.15*).

11.6 Can one do skin tests in children?

The key is cooperation: if the child is comfortable and compliant, then the tests are simple to do. However, if the child is agitated it will be impossible to keep the arm still enough to place the skin test solutions and prick them. In younger children, the number of skin tests should be kept to the minimum necessary to make a relevant diagnosis.

11.7 Are there any particular signs of allergic disease in children?

Allergic salute (*Fig. 11.2*); allergic facies; allergic nasal crease.

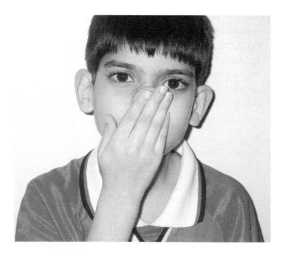

▲

Fig 11.2 'Allergy salute' is a characteristic sign of children with chronic allergic rhinitis. From Arshad SH 2002. Allergy: An Illustrated Colour Text Edinburgh: Churchill Livingstone, with permisson.

11.8 What should be done about allergies in school playgrounds?

Peanut allergy is becoming increasingly common among school-age children. Many parents of nut-allergic children are worried that their child may be accidentally exposed to nuts as a result of swapping snacks or sandwiches with playmates. Some schools have instituted nut-free policies for school meals and snacks; others have created special areas in their playgrounds where nut-allergic children are forced to spend their break time. As with most things in life, there is a balance to be struck. On the one hand, it is clearly inappropriate to isolate nut-allergic children from their peers unless there is overwhelming reason to do so. Most nut-allergic children have local swelling or urticaria from accidental exposure, and are not really at risk of death from inadvertent peanut ingestion. In areas where skin testing is freely available, a significant proportion of those labelled as peanut-allergic have positive skin tests without any clear history of allergic reactions. It is debatable whether these children really need to avoid nuts, and certainly one would not want to impose draconian restrictions on their play.

11.9 Which snacks are best to avoid an allergic reaction?

Accidental exposure to nuts is more likely with unknown foods and processed snacks than with material that is familiar or home-produced. Nut-allergic children should be encouraged to try a variety of food at home, but to be more conservative when visiting other houses and parties.

11.10 Is it dangerous to kiss people who have eaten peanuts?

Some nut-allergic children are extremely sensitive and can react even to the touch of a nut. This group may react to the traces of nut carried on the lips of someone who has eaten nuts. Clearly the risk of such contamination varies according to the individual family's custom and practice of greeting and familiarity.

11.11 How can a child be kept safe without making them stand out from the crowd?

Talk to the class teacher. Most teachers are familiar with the problems, and most schools will have policies in place to deal with asthma and food allergies. Local paediatricians will often have advice packs for schools and for parents of allergic children. Further information may be obtained from Allergy UK (see Appendix).

11.12 How should children with egg or milk allergy be managed?

See Question 9.24.

11.13 Is goat or sheep milk an acceptable substitute in patients with cow's milk allergy?

See Question 9.25.

11.14 Should children with cow's milk allergy be rechallenged and, if so, when?

See Question 9.26.

PROGNOSIS

11.15 Do children really grow out of their asthma?

Wheeze before the age of 3 years is primarily driven by the size of the airways, with those affected having small airways which give audible wheezing when the child contracts viral infections such as respiratory syncytial virus. This is only randomly associated with the subsequent development of asthma. Of course, some children will continue to have wheeze because they started with small airways and also inherited the tendency to allergic sensitization. Among those who develop asthma in childhood, most will lose their symptoms by the age of 18 years. Approximately 30% will continue with asthma into adulthood, while a proportion of those who lose their asthma in their teenage years will eventually experience a recurrence as they grow older. Factors associated with persistence of asthma include early age of onset, severity of asthma and female sex. The benefit of early and thorough treatment is not known, but it is hoped that prompt and effective anti-asthma therapy may minimize the long-term consequences of the disease.

THE FUTURE

11.16 How can we prevent future generations of children from developing allergies?

A million dollar question to which we do not have any definite answers. The main approaches are:

■ to define the factors responsible for developing allergy and asthma
■ to search for therapies that will prevent progression from atopy to asthma
■ to search for therapies that will accelerate the rate and frequency of remission from asthma.

11.17 How can pregnant women reduce the risk of their unborn child developing allergies?

The most crucial period for allergy prevention is from birth to 1 year. However, some forward planning is helpful and there are measures to take both before becoming pregnant and during the pregnancy itself.

11.18 What measures can be taken before becoming pregnant?

Stop smoking — this advice is highly pertinent as smoking has many ill effects in pregnancy and on the unborn child: increasing the risk of allergies is just one of them.

Plan the timing of the child's birth — being born just before or during the pollen season increases the risk of seasonal allergic rhinitis. The effect is strongest for tree pollens but it may also apply for grasses. Babies are most at risk from sensitization during their first 3–6 months of life.

Reduce damp from natural causes or from newly laid concrete or plaster as damp promotes the growth of moulds and house dust mite. For babies expected in the winter a dehumidifier to keep the moisture down may be advisable.

11.19 How can parents help prevent a child developing allergies?

Breast feed for at least 4 months, preferably 6 months; avoid early weaning; and especially avoid egg and cow's milk before 4 months. Avoid passive smoking, especially from the mother. Keep pets out of the bedroom, and minimize the level of dust in the child's bedroom by reducing clutter, and choosing hard flooring or removable rugs rather than fitted carpets.

PATIENT QUESTIONS

11.20 What can I do during pregnancy to reduce the chance of my child developing allergies?

Smoking during pregnancy is a clear cut risk factor for allergy. Maternal diet is not a major factor, although some doctors recommend that atopic mothers should not eat peanuts during pregnancy (to reduce the risk of their baby becoming sensitized, although there is no hard proof that this makes any difference).

Do not take metoprolol (Betaloc, Co-betaloc, Lopressor and Lopresoretic) during pregnancy. This drug is thought to increase the risk of allergies in children if taken by their mothers while pregnant. Comparable data on other beta-blockers are not available.

Antihistamines are not recommended during pregnancy, but there is little hard data to support this recommendation. Antihistamines do cause problems in lactating mothers: they are concentrated in the breast milk and may thus be transferred in higher than desirable dose to breast-fed babies.

Avoid major household renovations as these stir up house dust mite and mould spores. If unavoidable clean up very carefully.

Measures to be taken during pregnancy:
The most important thing to do at this stage is to reduce the allergens in the home. Specific things to consider are:

- Ensuring the baby's mattress and bedding is free from mite allergens
- Reducing animal allergens
- Reducing damp in the house
- Developing a smoke-free house
- Preparing to breast feed.

On current evidence there is no need for expectant mothers to avoid any allergens whilst pregnant. Whilst some babies can become sensitized in the womb to foods eaten by the mother this is such a rare and unusual event that it does not justify putting pregnant women on special diets.
As discussed above, aim to breast feed for 4–6 months if possible. Wean slowly and not too early.

11.21 Are pets really a risk for allergies and asthma?

In general, pets are risk factors for the development of asthma and should be avoided by those with atopic pedigrees. Allowing pets in the bedrooms is a bad idea (whether occasional visits by cats or a resident rodent). The safest pets are fish or 'adopted' animals at the local zoo.

11.22 What should I do if my child is allergic to our pets?

When children are found to be allergic to pets, it can be a very difficult decision to part with the pet. To quote one distraught parent 'my children will leave home but pets are for life'. Possible options include confining the pet to the kitchen where it is easier to clean, donating the pet to grandparents or friends so that occasional visits are possible, or finding another home for the pet. It should be noted that cat allergens in particular are extremely persistent in the environment and it can take 6 months or more before the level of cat allergens reverts to background. Cat allergens can also persist in soft furnishings for many months, so the benefits of removing the pet can be less than anticipated unless thorough cleaning is undertaken.

11.23 What are the recommendations for vaccination in an allergic child?

Generally this is not a problem, but caution is required if a child has a true allergy to hen's eggs. Some MMR vaccines contain traces of egg protein which in rare instances can cause an allergic reaction. You should ensure that your doctor is made aware of any allergy to eggs and checks that the vaccine to be used is egg-free.

If there is a history of egg allergy producing severe symptoms, and it is necessary to give a vaccine containing egg protein, the correct procedure is referral to hospital. The allergic child can then undergo skin prick testing to the vaccine before immunization. If no response occurs immunization can proceed. If the child is sensitized to components of the vaccine, it may be possible to find an alternative source of vaccine; otherwise a judgement has to be made on a case by case basis of the risks to the child of vaccination *versus* the risks of non-vaccination.

11.24 When is it safe to start to give peanut butter to children?

Nobody knows for sure, but in children with atopic parents, it is probably best to avoid it completely before the age of 6 months and, arguably, the longer you delay the less likely the child is to become allergic to peanuts.

11.25 What factors should be considered if asthma appears to be associated with school?

School-associated asthma may be caused by a number of different factors. Probably the commonest is exercise-induced wheeze, which is common in all asthmatics. Children who experience this should be encouraged to be active and to participate in sports to the best of their ability. Swimming is often easier than outdoor sports, as the impact of hyperventilation on the irritable airway is less when the air is warm and damp.

Complementary therapy

INTRODUCTION

12.1 Why are people with allergies particularly interested in alternative medicine (complementary medicine)?

Conventional allergy practice is not beyond criticism. Patients often experience difficulties in obtaining clear and helpful advice from the healthcare system, either because they are a long way from sources of information or because the information that is available is not appropriate to their particular needs. Sometimes their GP is unaware of the allergy services provided. Whatever the reason, it is not unusual for patients concerned about allergy to feel lacking in the help and support they need. Patients' willingness to explore new therapies may be further accentuated by the chronicity of their condition, the inadequacy of conventional pharmacotherapy and the impracticalities of allergen avoidance. Conventional medicine appears to offer ways of containing the condition rather than curing it, so alternative cures seem an attractive option. Other patients believe that conventional medications are harmful, and so they look for ways to reduce the amount of medication, especially when it is a corticosteroid.

12.2 What do alternative practitioners mean when they say 'allergy'?

It is hard to generalize, but most alternative therapists use the term allergic in the lay sense — as in 'I'm allergic to Monday mornings' — rather than in the medical or scientific sense of there being immune recognition of a foreign substance that in turn causes an allergic reaction. Patients are often told they are 'allergic' to substances and should reduce their intake, rather than avoid them completely as one would with the conventional use of the term. Increasingly, alternative therapists use the term 'intolerant' instead of allergic. While this may be a more accurate description of the clinical entity, it does not mean that the tests being used to diagnose intolerance have any greater validity than those being used to recognize allergy incorrectly.

12.3 Do alternative therapists treating allergy have an evidence base for their work?

The evidence base for the role of alternative therapies in allergic diseases is extremely limited. It must be assumed that alternative therapists believe in the validity of what they are doing, otherwise they would be guilty of fraud. However, there are undoubtedly some alternative therapists who are taking patients for a ride. In this sense they are no better or worse than palm-readers or fortune-tellers, both of which are perfectly legal. From a purely factual point of view there is no evidence that any of the electrical, physical, reflex or analytical techniques offered have any value in diagnosing trigger factors for allergic conditions.

Interestingly, the advice given by alternative therapists to all patients with allergic conditions is similar, with the diagnosis and management being based more on the history than the results of any 'tests'.

12.4 Are there ever disputes between conventional and alternative therapists regarding the management of allergic patients?

Sometimes patients may come to grief by preferring the advice of an alternative practitioner. For example, the peanut-allergic child whose parents are reassured on non-conventional testing that the nut allergy has resolved, but the uncontrolled reintroduction of peanuts into the diet precipitates an anaphylactic reaction. Following these unhappy incidents there are often interesting and lively discussions but little beyond this. If, for example, a conventional practitioner accused an alternative therapist of practising fraudulently, the onus would be on the accuser to prove that the alternative therapist did not believe in what they are saying. Accusations that the alternative therapist is damaging the patient would be based on the financial contract between the patient and the therapist, so the opinion of the conventional practitioner is irrelevant unless the patient thinks there is a problem or the practitioner is registered with a professional body such as the General Medical Council in the UK. (The concept of negligence is needed in the UK in NHS practice to deal with the situation where the practitioner and the patient do not have a direct contract, because no money changes hands.)

12.5 Does mercury in dental amalgam cause allergies?

There is no evidence that it does. A number of patients have been concerned that they may be poisoned by the mercury in dental amalgam and that the mercury may adversely affect their immune system. Some dentists make a living removing 'unnatural' mercury fillings and replacing them with 'natural' plastic and resin. The total lifetime exposure to mercury from a full set of amalgam fillings is less than 1% of the maximal permissible exposure limit for mercury. There is no evidence that heavy metal poisoning can occur at this level of exposure, or that this level of mercury exposure has any effect on the immune system or on the body's ability to tolerate other substances.

12.6 Does *Candida* cause allergies?

Candida albicans is a yeast that grows on all our bodies. It does not usually cause disease, but can cause local irritation in the mouth, vagina and other moist areas, especially if the local defence mechanisms are impaired, for example, by topical steroids or by diabetes mellitus. *Candida* does not invade the body except when T lymphocytes are seriously compromised (e.g. in advanced cancer, in AIDS and in patients taking immunosuppressive drugs for transplantation, cancer, autoimmune disease, etc.). Almost everyone shows T cell responses to *Candida* (this is used as a routine test of the integrity of the immune system), and some will also show antibodies directed against *Candida*, but there is no convincing evidence that hypersensitivity to *Candida* causes or contributes to any human illnesses.

12.7 Why is it important to enquire about alternative therapies when taking an allergy history?

This additional question will help you to understand the patient's medical and philosophical approach to their allergy. However, very few of the treatments interact with, or have any bearing on, the choice of conventional therapy.

A whole raft of alternative therapies and natural remedies are being used by patients to manage their allergies (*Box 12.1*), and sometimes it may be necessary to probe and prompt to obtain the full picture.

BOX 12.1 Alternative treatments and natural remedies frequently used to treat allergic disorders

Acupuncture
Alexander technique
Aromatherapy
Bach flower remedies
Herbalism
Homeopathy
Hydrotherapy
Hypnotherapy
Massage
Naturopathy
Reflexology

DIAGNOSIS

12.8 Should any notice be taken of the VEGA tests my patient has obtained and now brings to my attention?

Basically no, but you should listen to the patient's reasons for seeking such tests and it is necessary to debrief them on the nature of the test that was done and validity of the advice given.

The VEGA test, abbreviated from 'vegetative reflex test' is claimed to measure the concentration of certain compounds within the body or the body's reactivity towards the test substances. The test is performed differently by different practitioners, but some common aspects can be identified. The practitioner connects the patient to the machine by electrodes, which are placed at various sites on the body, usually acupuncture points related to the patient's condition. The practitioner then inserts a glass vial containing a dilution of one or more test substances into a metal honeycomb that forms part of the electrical circuit. The practitioner tells the patient what is being tested and then records any change in the electrical measurement. The device is usually calibrated on a 100-point scale, taking zero as safe (distilled water) and 100 as the maximum 'disorder' reading (e.g. with a dilution of Paraquat or other harmful substance). A series of vials containing different substances is then tested. Most readings from this device fall in the 40–60 range, and the practitioner puts an arbitrary cut-off of 50 for recording something as relevant. The patient is given a form listing the substances tested and those to which they showed a response.

12.9 If not assessing allergic status, what does a VEGA test measure?

From a conventional perspective, the electrical device is a Wheatstone bridge, which measures the resistance across the patient's skin. When the patient is tested against something they consider harmful, the electrical resistance of the skin decreases and so the device measures a change. This test is similar to a form of lie detector. There is no evidence whatsoever that the vials emit bioradiation (as claimed by alternative practitioners) and so the stimulus to alterations in skin resistance would appear to be the naming of substances as the vial is put in and out of the device. Where the substances are not named, the readings appear to be random. A recent evaluation of VEGA testing found that the test was unable to detect allergy to cats or house dust mite in patients who were proven to have allergies by standard blood and skin tests.

12.10 What other tests are being used by complementary therapists and is there any evidence to support their accuracy?

As well as VEGA tests, there are a variety of equally implausible tests in use. These include:

- Applied kinesiology, where the patient is given a vial to hold and the practitioner tests the power of the free arm.
- Variations in which the vial containing the test substance is placed over the affected organ (chest, nose, abdomen, etc.) and arm power is tested.
- Auriculocardiac reflex — the practitioner applies a drop of the test substance to the ear lobe and feels the pulse to see whether the pulse rate increases transiently in response to the test substance.

■ Hair analysis — usually for trace minerals, but this is sometimes claimed to be useful in diagnosing allergies.

■ Leukocytotoxic tests — a small amount of test substance is incubated with the patient's cells on a slide: the effects of the test substance are assessed by microscopic examination of the visual appearance of the white blood cells.

■ Provocation–neutralization tests — tiny amounts of a test substance are given as drops, subcutaneous injections or intradermal injections, and the patient's responses are monitored (by peak flow rate, skin response, etc.). When there is a positive response, the dose used previously is called the provocation dose. The dose is then reduced until the response ceases. This is then called the neutralization dose and is used for therapy.

MANAGEMENT

12.11 Is there any clinical evidence that complementary approaches work and, if so, which techniques work for which allergies?

Without exception, complementary diagnostic techniques are without value, but some of the management advice given by complementary practitioners is both sensible and helpful. For example, most patients with irritable bowel syndrome (IBS) will improve if they reduce their intake of wheat and/or cow's milk. Almost every patient with IBS who consults an alternative practitioner will be given this advice, but the tests done to demonstrate that they may react to the food have no bearing on the validity of the advice.

Providing patients with something they can do to help regain control of their lives is usually beneficial. This is true whether it is a treatment (homeopathic drops, dietary supplements, etc.) or lifestyle advice (diets, advice on stress management, etc.). Reducing intake of caffeine and alcohol can make people feel better in themselves, especially if their consumption of these drugs is a response to stress in their lives. Provided the advice and therapy proposed is harmless and does not lead to bankruptcy, there is no conflict with conventional therapy.

Many alternative therapies purport to boost the body's immune system so that the allergens can be destroyed, to counteract the symptoms by the use of natural antihistamines and to keep the body 'in balance' and stress-free. Whilst the efficacy of many of these approaches on the immune system or on the clinical conditions is not proven, we have to recognize that the therapies may have wide appeal to patients. An important part of our role is to ensure that patients obtain objective advice when they ask for it, and do not expose themselves unknowingly to harmful products.

12.12 Can essential oils help treat allergic conditions?

Most major chemists and health stores stock aromatherapy oils, of which many are recommended for hay fever (*Box 12.2*). The oils may bring symptomatic relief when used in the bath or in a steam inhalation.

BOX 12.2 Essential oils recommended for hay fever

Boswellia thurifera (frankincense)
Cedrus libani (cedarwood)
Cymbopogon nardus (citronella) as a steam inhalation
Eucalyptus globulus (eucalyptus) — decongestant used in the bath or as a steam inhalation or as a massage oil. A drop on the pillow may reduce night-time stuffiness
Illcium anisatum (aniseed) as a steam inhalation or as a massage for the chest and back to loosen mucus and relieve sinusitis
Matricaria recutita (camomile) — recommended for its calming and soothing properties
Rosa (rose) — its anti-inflammatory and mildly sedative properties in the bath are said to aid relaxation and improve breathing
Thymus vulgaris (thyme) — renowned for its ability to relieve congestion and ease breathing difficulties. Should be used as a massage for the chest and back or in a steam inhalation

---

12.13 Can people become allergic to essential oils?

Essential oils used in aromatherapy are highly concentrated and can cause allergic skin reactions if not correctly diluted. For massage the oils require diluting with massage oil in the proportions two drops of aromatherapy oil to 5 ml massage oil. Camomile is best avoided by patients allergic to ragweed as there is a risk of a cross-reaction.

12.14 Are there any natural treatments to unblock the nose in rhinitis?

The traditional treatments used for colds, saline nasal drops and steam inhalation, can also bring symptom relief in hay fever and rhinitis. The addition of menthol, eucalyptus or other aromatic substances (*Question 12.12*) to the steam inhalation improves its effect. These can be bought as essential oils or in capsule form (e.g. Karvol®). Steam inhalation can be low-tech (e.g. leaning over a bowl with a towel over the head) or using a commercial device which supplies a continuous stream of warm moist air. When tested with individuals suffering from the common cold it achieved superior relief of symptoms than a conventional steam inhalation, but its efficacy in hay fever has not been tested.

12.15 Are dietary supplements useful for hay fever sufferers?

Extrapolating from other diseases, fish oils such as cod liver oil (two teaspoons daily) may be beneficial in hay fever. Fish oils affect the production of prostaglandins and reduce the tendency for inflammation in the body. This is of proven benefit in rheumatoid arthritis and may also be valuable in asthma and hay fever. Evening primrose oil is likewise used for rheumatoid arthritis and may have a role to play in allergic disorders. Both cod liver oil and evening primrose oil take 3 months to exert their effects fully on prostaglandin production, and patients need to be encouraged to persist with treatment as to maintain any effect requires continuing dosing.

Other suggested dietary supplements are high-dose vitamin C, ginseng or cider vinegar, but there is no trial evidence of effectiveness. An additional suggestion is honey from locally produced honeycomb; this is proposed as it contains pollen and, whilst its effectiveness has never been formally tested, it would seem unlikely to work as the pollen in honey is rarely the sort to which hay fever sufferers react.

12.16 Does acupuncture help in asthma?

Within Chinese medicine acupuncture has been used to treat eczema, asthma and rhinitis. There is some evidence that acupuncture in asthma might work, but for rhinitis and eczema there is little more than anecdote. The lack of hard evidence may be interpreted by a sceptic as proof that it does not work, but a patient who has benefited would hold a strongly opposing view! Formal evaluation of acupuncture is awaited as it is generally a safe treatment and patients may wish to try it. It is important to realize that the effect will not be immediate as acupuncture works in stages. As the course of acupuncture treatments progress, so should the response to treatment improve. A course of treatments usually totals 4–10 sessions. If there has been no response with the first four treatments then acupuncture will probably prove to be ineffective in that patient. A common problem that can occur with acupuncture is a transitory worsening of symptoms or 'reaction' after treatment. Such a reaction will resolve over a few days and, interestingly, its presence usually indicates that this particular patient will later respond to treatment.

Acupuncture is relatively free from serious side-effects providing the needles are sterilized and disposed of after use. Needle insertion may frighten some people and cause them to faint. The insertion of the needles may be uncomfortable, but is rarely painful. Occasionally, bruising at the site of insertion is observed.

12.17 What advice should be given to patients with eczema who wish to use Chinese herbal remedies?

Some patients with eczema seem to benefit. Unlike homeopathy and other low-dose regimes, Chinese herbal medicines contain a variety of very active drugs. Some of the 'herbs' have been adulterated with corticosteroids which would help to explain why they work in eczema!

Some of these preparations can damage the liver and such concerns have reduced their popularity. A more minor consideration is that some patients may find the taste of the preparations unpalatable. Probably the most appropriate response to your patient's request is to consult with your local dermatologist about the emerging evidence and reputable remedies.

12.18 Are there any dangers of complementary therapy in the treatment of allergies?

Several problems come to mind:

- Some natural remedies do in fact contain pharmacologically active substances which may have unexpected or predictable side-effects. As the medicine is not prepared or regulated in the same way as conventional medicines, the patient and any other attending physicians may not realize that side-effects are caused by the complementary medicine.
- The patient may be advised or may decide for themselves to drop other parts of their treatment regime. For rhinitis this is not a big deal, but for asthma and other serious conditions it can put the patient at risk.
- The patient may become dependent on the therapist and, where money changes hands, there is a risk that the therapist may not wish to let the patient stand on their own feet because that compromises the therapist's income.
- The patient may find that they feel better but they cannot afford to continue the therapy. In the UK, the NHS is generally unwilling to foot the bill, and this can lead to conflict between the patient and their GP, who is seen as acting on behalf of the NHS system rather than on behalf of the patient. Naturally the reality is somewhere in between, as the GP has a responsibility to the patient, but also has to balance the costs and benefits of therapy against the legitimate demands of others on the healthcare budget.

THE FUTURE

12.19 What are the future needs for alternative therapy?

To assess the claims made for complementary and alternative allergy techniques, a set of agreed case definitions must be established, especially for those conditions that conventional allergists do not consider to be allergic in nature. The current haphazard use of diagnostic methods needs harmonizing and validating. Any worthwhile diagnostic method should work equally well whoever is using it and wherever it is being used. Similarly, it should be possible to standardize treatments so that patients with similar clinical problems who show similar test results receive the same therapeutic approach. If personality and other unconventional aspects are important in deciding on a therapy, it should be possible to codify this in some way that is transparent, and not simply dependent on the whim of the therapist. Formal assessment is required of the usefulness of unconventional diagnostic and therapeutic techniques using objective assessments of outcome, and ideally these should be compared with the best available conventional treatment.

PATIENT QUESTIONS

12.20 What is enzyme-potentiated desensitization?

In this technique, a very small amount of allergen (about one-hundredth of what would be given in standard immunotherapy) is given by injection together with a dose of the enzyme beta-galactosidase. The theory behind the therapy is that the beta-galactosidase alters the way that the allergen is handled in the body, so that the effect of the tiny amount of allergen is potentiated, and it becomes as effective as standard doses of immunotherapy without carrying the same risk of side-effects. This is a laudable aim, but has never been properly proven, either at the basic or clinical level. Enzyme-potentiated desensitization thus remains a fringe treatment, available only in unconventional allergy services.

12.21 My local chemist sells a homeopathic hay fever remedy. Should I try it?

Homeopathy is a form of treatment developed by a German doctor, Samuel Hahnemann, at the end of the 18th century. It is based on the idea that like cures like and uses substances that produce the same symptoms as those it aims to treat. The substance used is called a similium and this is diluted repeatedly before being used in the preparation of tablets. Homeopathy developed a good reputation as it was far pleasanter and safer than the horrible procedures (such as bloodletting, cathartics and emetics) being promulgated by Hahnemann's colleagues. However, if one examines the scientific basis for this treatment it is impossible to produce an explanation of why a 'dilution' that is so weak that it does not contain any of the original similium can bestow healing properties.

It then becomes difficult for anyone to recommend or justify the purchase of such a remedy.

If you visit a homeopath rather than buying an over-the-counter remedy from your chemist, you will also experience a long consultation with a sympathetic therapist who will be able to answer your questions and provide advice. You may well benefit more from this whole-person or holistic approach rather than taking the medication in isolation, but the cost will be considerably more.

12.22 What should I consider when choosing a complementary therapist?

- Qualifications and experience
- Are they registered with a governing body?
- Reputation and personal recommendations
- Is the therapist happy to communicate with your GP?
- What does the treatment involve (frequency, duration, cost)?

Be cautious of the therapist who promises to 'cure' you of your allergy or discourages you from taking your conventional medication. Acute attacks of asthma and anaphylaxis should always be managed with conventional treatments and by qualified doctors.

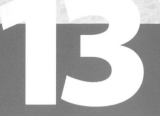

Travel and allergy

INTRODUCTION

13.1 Why are the allergy services of Europe and North America organized so differently from the UK service?

The NHS in the UK is primarily organized around organ-based specialities, like cardiology, respiratory medicine, dermatology, etc. There are a few exceptions (e.g. diabetes) but mechanisms-based disciplines tend to be confined to academic departments. This contrasts with North America and most European countries, where allergy is a mainstream hospital speciality, with equivalent standing to the organ-based specialities. Indeed, in the US, people with asthma would normally expect to see an allergist first and would only go to see a chest doctor if they failed to make progress with their allergist. France is an exception, with allergy mainly practised by primary care doctors with a certificate of competence in allergy. Allergy developed as a freestanding speciality in the US during the 1930s, but in the UK, the diagnosis and treatment of allergic conditions was largely confined to general practice until 1986 when regulations were introduced to restrict the delivery of immunotherapy in primary care. This decision led to the allergen manufacturers withdrawing from the UK market, as they felt it was not worthwhile to continue to market skin test solutions for allergy diagnosis if they could not sell their vaccines for immunotherapy. Allergy continued in academic units, which had always been interested in the mechanisms of disease, but there were insufficient of these to provide a diagnostic and therapeutic service across the whole UK.

The financial frameworks of individual healthcare systems have also influenced the development of allergy services. In the UK, the system of universal provision with salaried hospital staff (known in the US as socialized medicine) has had a profound effect on the development of hospital-based services. In general, hospitals have focused on major life-threatening illnesses and disorders affecting the elderly, but have been unresponsive to public demand for better care for disorders that are seen as inconvenient but not life-threatening. Hence the UK's poor performance on elective surgery, conservative dentistry, etc. Unfortunately, allergic conditions have often been regarded as unimportant by hospital management committees, and hence there has been a reluctance to train and appoint staff to deal with allergic disorders. In Europe, where most countries have social insurance systems, patients have demanded and largely have received care for the conditions that trouble them most, including allergies. Under their fee-for-service reimbursement schemes, there have been substantial incentives for physicians to increase their workload and provide allergy care for more and more people. Under these differing regimes, custom and practice have evolved differently in different countries, and this variation is more marked in allergy than it is in some other 'mainstream' specialities such as cardiology or respiratory medicine.

13.2   Which allergens are important in different countries?

Seasonal and climatic differences have profound effects on the pollen calendar in different countries. In Northern Europe, birch pollen is a major problem, while grass pollen is a short-lived, late-summer phenomenon. In the Mediterranean, the grass pollen season is over by Easter, but there are major problems with *Parietaria*, which has a prolonged flowering season from February to October, varying a bit depending on the precise location. In the US, ragweed is a major problem, causing an autumn hay fever season.

Indoor allergens also vary from country to country. House dust mites are happiest in damp temperate climates, but other mites flourish in hotter damp climates. On the US eastern seaboard, house dust mite is a major problem in middle class homes with air conditioning, but cockroach is the dominant allergen in low-rent housing. At altitudes above 1000 metres, house dust mites are rarely found, but people still develop allergies. In Arizona, for example, there is almost no allergy to house dust mites, but many children are allergic to dogs. In this area, dogs are kept indoors (apparently they risk being eaten by coyotes if they are left outside at night) and so there are very high levels of dog allergens in Arizona homes.

13.3   Do people's allergies change when they move from one country to another to live?

When allergic people move to live in another country, they often experience a honeymoon period, with little or no symptoms for the first 2 years. Afterwards, they often show signs of sensitization to the major local allergens (e.g. ragweed in the US, grass pollen in the UK). Those who are sensitized to allergens found in both countries may find that the pattern of their symptoms alters. For example, house dust mite allergen levels are pretty constant over the year in the UK, but in the US these levels vary markedly over the year because of the much greater seasonal changes in humidity and temperature.

DIAGNOSIS

13.4   Are the same methods used for diagnosis in different countries?

Within mainstream allergy practice, the approach is similar, with skin testing used to back up the diagnosis made on the history. Some countries prefer to perform skin tests on the back rather than on the arm; some prefer intradermal skin tests rather than the skin prick tests used in the UK. Unconventional tests for allergy diagnosis vary from practitioner to practitioner and are outside the scope of this chapter.

MANAGEMENT

13.5 Do treatment strategies vary from country to country?

The basic principles of allergy diagnosis and treatment are shared. The allergist tries to identify trigger factors and provide advice on avoiding or minimizing exposure. The choice of anti-allergic drugs and anti-asthma drugs does vary according to local custom and experience, as well as with the availability of newer medications. Compared to other developed countries, UK practice is reluctant to use immunotherapy, especially in patients with asthma.

13.6 What advice and treatment should allergic patients be given before travelling abroad?

Those on regular medication need to take adequate supplies of their anti-allergic medication with them and also a written record of what they use in case of loss. The general precaution of travelling with one's medication in hand luggage avoids the additional hassle of obtaining replacement medication should the luggage for the hold go astray. Whilst good data is available on pollen levels and seasons elsewhere, occasionally unusual weather conditions can shift the season by several weeks, so even if the patient is in search of a pollen-free break they should, as a precaution, take their anti-allergic medication.

13.7 Is one allowed to take an Epipen on an aircraft?

Under current anti-terrorist regulations, syringes with needles are only allowed on aircraft in hand baggage if the passenger can provide documentation that they may need to use the equipment on the flight. Airlines recognize that food allergy (*see Question 9.49*) and anaphylaxis are sound reasons for bringing emergency equipment on to the plane, and will allow Epipens to be carried on aircraft provided the carrier has a letter from their GP or specialist explaining that they have a serious allergy and need to carry their Epipen with them at all times (*see Question 6.20*).

13.8 What generic advice should be given to patients with house dust mite allergy about choosing a holiday destination?

Most patients would prefer their atopic problems to be no worse and preferably better when on holiday. Therefore advice should include avoiding old or damp accommodation, and thinking twice about properties close to water. Going at the beginning of the season to a property that has been unused for many months may be particularly troublesome. Taking one's own sleeping bag and/or microporous pillow covers, duvet covers and mattress covers can help minimize exposure to mites in bed. Mountains, for example the Alps, make an ideal destination as mites are not found above 2000 metres.

13.9 If patients want to identify the pollen counts in advance of travelling where can they look?

Information is available from:

- Telephone help lines
- Books
- Specialized pollen advice services.

Telephone help lines offer information on the pollen count (from the previous day), the forecast for the day and often the outlook for the next 3 days. People needing more specialized information about distant locations can often find details in self-help books such as *The Complete Guide to Hayfever* by Jonathon Brostoff and Linda Gamlin (Paragon Publishing, 1998). More detailed advice may be available by writing to regional or national aeroallergen research centres.

13.10 In our travel clinic patients often ask about suitable sunscreens as they react to various products — what advice should be given?

When travelling to hot climes there is no alternative to taking protection from both UVA and UVB. Allergy to sunscreen is uncommon; most adverse reactions are either irritant, a polymorphic light eruption or prickly heat. Occasionally, patients may have urticaria triggered by sunlight.

Rather than experiment with different sunscreens patients may be tempted to tolerate sunburn, but this should be discouraged. Explaining that sunscreens are much less likely to cause sensitization now than in the past may help. Previously they used to contain high concentrations of one agent, but now they contain low concentrations of three or four agents to minimize the risk of allergy. Sunscreens may be mistakenly labelled as 'hypoallergenic' because they contain no PABA, but of course they may contain other potentially problematic chemical agents. Similarly 'natural' is not synonymous with safe. If the patient cannot identify a suitable product by trial and error, then formal patch testing to identify the offending substances may be appropriate. If referral for patch testing is not easy and true sunscreen allergy is suspected, an alternative option is a physical sunscreen. These non-chemical sunblockers act by physically blocking light rays from the skin. Titanium dioxide and zinc oxide are commonly used, but people may dislike their opaque appearance.

Generic advice on suncare strategies (clothing, sunglasses, hat, regular reapplication of sunblock, etc.) should obviously accompany the above.

PATIENT QUESTIONS

13.11 Will my allergies get better or worse when I go on holiday?

Most patients will find improvement if they go abroad on holiday.
Those with hay fever may avoid the grass pollen season, which typically
happens in March in the Mediterranean, and few will be sensitized to the
pollens that cause trouble in the Mediterranean basin (e.g. olive, *Parietaria*,
etc.). Similarly, people with house dust mite allergy will generally find that
the drier climate of the Mediterranean will mean reduced exposure to the
allergen responsible for driving their symptoms. Different considerations
apply in other parts of the world. House dust mite is mainly a problem in
damp temperate climates while pollen seasons vary according to latitude.

13.12 I worry about not being able to explain my child's allergy in another language. What can I do?

Patient support organizations such as Allergy UK offer a series of translation
cards that are available in most European languages. These cards carry
messages which describe the allergy, request food without the allergen, or
ask for medical help. The cards are laminated, with English on one side and
the foreign translation on the reverse.

When preparing for a holiday don't forget also to check the healthcare
cover included in your travel insurance.

13.13 Can people be allergic to tropical fruit?

Yes. Quite a lot of people are allergic to bananas. This may be an isolated
problem, or may be due to a cross-reaction with latex. Many patients with
latex allergy react to several different tropical fruits, including bananas,
mango, and papaya (paw-paw), because there are similar proteins in these
fruit and in latex. The same proteins are also found in sweet chestnuts (also
known as Spanish or edible chestnuts). Anyone who is allergic to these fruits
should avoid them, but should also be assessed for possible latex allergy.

APPENDIX
Useful organisations

Charities, patient organisations and support groups

ACTION AGAINST ALLERGY
PO Box 278
Twickenham TW1 4QQ
Tel: 020 8892 4949/2711
Fax: 020 8892 4950

http://www.actionagainstallergy.co.uk/

UK charity which aims to advance understanding, awareness and recognition of allergic medical conditions and allergy-related illness, and the actions needed for research, diagnosis and treatment. Offers information packs and leaflets on a wide range of allergy subjects, including non-allergenic products, and details of local allergy clinics.

ALLERGY UK (OPERATIONAL NAME FOR THE BRITISH ALLERGY FOUNDATION)
Deepdene House
30 Bellegrove Road
Welling
Kent DA16 3PY
Tel: 020 8303 8525
Fax: 020 8303 8792
Helpline: 020 8303 8583 (Monday to Friday, 9.00am–5.00pm)

http://www.allergyfoundation.com/

Provides information, advice and support for people with allergies. Lists NHS allergy clinics and the specialists involved, and products of practical help to people with allergies. Has local support groups.

NATIONAL ASTHMA CAMPAIGN
National Asthma Campaign
Providence House
Providence Place
London N1 0NT
Tel: 020 7226 2260
Helpline: 0845 7 01 02 03 (Monday to Friday, 9.00am–7.00pm)
Fax: 020 7704 0740

http://www.asthma.org.uk/

UK charity working in partnership with people with asthma and all who share their concern, through research, education and support. Offers factsheets online, and a telephone helpline for sufferers. Publishes booklets, leaflets and videos (including videos on self-management of asthma in several Asian languages.

ASTHMA SOCIETY OF IRELAND
Eden House
15–17 Eden Quay
Dublin, 1
Ireland
Phone: +353 1 878 8511
Asthma Line: +353 1850 44 54 64
Liveline: +35 1 8788122 (Monday and Friday, 9.30am–1.00pm, Thursday, 9.30am–5.30pm).
Fax: +353 1 878 8128
Email: asthma@indigo.ie

http://www.asthmasociety.ie/

Provides information, advice and reassurance to people with asthma and their families, acts as advocate/representative for them, and promotes awareness and understanding of the condition amongst the general public. Pre-recorded 24 hour Asthma Line, and Asthma LiveLine staffed by specialist trained nurses.

ASTHMA & ALLERGY FOUNDATION OF AMERICA (AAFA)
1233 20th Street, NW
Suite 402
Washington, D.C. 20036
Tel: 202.466.7643
Fax: 202.466.8940

http://www.aafa.org

US patient organization dedicated to improving the quality of life for people with asthma and allergies and their caregivers, through education, advocacy and research. Provides practical information, community based services, support and referrals through a national network of chapters and educational support groups. Also sponsors research toward better treatments and a cure for asthma and allergic diseases.

ASTHMA VICTORIA
69 Flemington Road, Nth Melbourne
VIC 3051
Tel: (03) 9326 7088
Toll Free helpline: 1800 645 130
Fax: (03) 9326 7055
Email: girving@asthma.org.au

http://www.asthma.org.au/events.htm

Offers education, advice, research and support, and runs events to raise awareness.

PEAK
Providence House
Providence Place
London N1 0NT
Tel: 020 7704 5892

http://www.asthma.org.uk/peakhome.html

Organises medically supported holidays in specialised centres for children aged 6–17 who have asthma and/or eczema. Run by the National Asthma Campaign.

NATIONAL ECZEMA SOCIETY
Hill House
Highgate Hill
London
N19 5NA
Tel: 020 7281 3553
Fax: 020 7281 6395
Helpline: 0870 241 3604 (Monday to Friday, 1.00pm–4.00pm)

http://www.eczema.org/

UK organisation for people with eczema, dermatitis and sensitive skin. Offers advice and support, represents patient views and funds research to identify causes and potential cures.

ECZEMA ASSOCIATION OF AUSTRALIA
Supports and educates eczema sufferers and carers, along with the wider community.

http://www.eczema.org.au/

PSORIASIS ASSOCIATION (UK)

Milton House
7 Milton Street
Northampton
NN2 7JG
Tel: 01604 711 129
Fax: 01604 792894

http://www.skincarecampaign.org/

Self-help organisation providing support and information to sufferers, carers, health professionals and others.

LATEX ALLERGY SUPPORT GROUP (UK)

102 Monkseaton Drive
Whitley Bay
Tyne & Wear NE26 3DJ
Tel/Fax: 0191 251 5432
Helpline: 07071 225838 (Every day, 7.00pm–10.00pm)

http://www.lasg.co.uk/

Information and support for people with a latex allergy. Include a list of everyday items that may contain latex and safe alternatives.

SKINSHIP

C/o Ashley Medicks
Plascow Cottage
Kirkgunzeon
Dumfries
DG2 8JT
Helpline: 01387 760 567

http://www.ukselfhelp.info/skinship/

Patient self-help and support group for sufferers of all types of skin conditions.

ANAPHYLAXIS CAMPAIGN

PO Box 275
Farnborough
Hampshire
GU14 6XS
Tel: 01252 542 029

http://www.anaphylaxis.org.uk/

UK charity aiming to promote public awareness of anaphylaxis and to advance and publish research into the causes and care of it. Website includes specific guidance for GPs and health workers, dietitians, caterers and school and college staff, as well as those who suffer from the condition.

COELIAC UK
PO Box 220
High Wycombe
Buckinghamshire HP11 2HY
Tel: 01494 437278
Helpline: 0870 444 8804
Fax: 01494 474349

http://www.coeliac.co.uk/

Information and support services for people with coeliac disease, including a food list of gluten-free manufactured products. Also funds research and raises public awareness of coeliac disease.

IBS NETWORK (UK)
Northern General Hospital
Sheffield
S5 7AU
(All written enquiries must be accompanied by an SAE)
Email: penny@ibsnetwork.org.uk

http://www.ibsnetwork.org.uk/

UK patient-led charity which aims to inform, support, and educate those with IBS and their families and carers; and to raise public awareness of IBS.

FOOD ALLERGY AND ANAPHYLAXIS NETWORK (USA)
www.foodallergy.org

Raising public awareness and acting as a communication link between the patient and dietitians, nurses, physicians, representatives from government agencies, and the food and pharmaceutical industries. Supports research and produces information booklets as well as actively involved in education.

FOOD ALLERGY INITIATIVE (USA)
625 Madison Avenue, 11th Floor
New York, NY 10022
Tel: 212.527.5835
Fax: 212.527.5837
Email: info@foodallergyinitiative.org

http://www.foodallergyinitiative.org

Non-profit organization founded to raise funds toward the effective treatment and cure for food allergies.

MEDIC ALERT
1 Bridge Wharf
156 Caledonian Road
London N1 9UU
Tel: 020 7833 3034
Fax: 020 7278 0647

http://www.medicalert.org/

Supplies emergency identification bracelets and pendants.

Patient information sites

http://www.nhsdirect.nhs.uk/SelfHelp/conditions/allergies/allergies.asp

(Helpline: 0845 4647, 24 hours a day, 7 days per week)
NHS Direct – provides information on diseases, treatments, self-help and support groups, complaints procedures and availability of NHS services.

http://www.niaid.nih.gov/publications/allergies.htm

US National Institutes of Health factsheets and other publications on various allergies.

http://www.users.globalnet.co.uk/~aair/

Asthma and Allergy Information and Research, the website of the Leicester Branch of the Midlands Asthma and Allergy Research Association (MAARA). It offers web-based information and patient leaflets on allergies.

http://www.allergicchild.com/

Information, advice and suggestions for coping strategies. Also offers book recommendations and a forum for parents of allergic children to share experiences and support one another, search for local support groups (mainly US).

http://pollenuk.worc.ac.uk/Next.htm

National Pollen Research Unit, for information about pollen and hay fever, including daily pollen forecasts for the UK.

http://www.talkeczema.com/docs/aboutus.htm

Personal site with links to other support and network sites, books on eczema and other products for eczema sufferers.

http://www.eczemavoice.com/

Personal site with support network, tips and information, particularly for parents of children with eczema, and 'Smile, its only eczema' badges.

http://www.pslgroup.com/ASTHMA.HTM

Collection of news and newsgroups on asthma.

http://www.asthmalearninglab.com/

Information about the causes, symptoms and treatments of asthma for patients and healthcare professionals.

http://www.radix.net/~mwg/asthma-gen.html

News/discussion group on asthma.

http://www.aanma.org

Nonprofit US site with news updates, tips, FAQs on allergy and asthma, and facility to email questions to a qualified nurse.

http://www.pollenuk.co.uk

Website of the Pollen Research Unit, University College. Worcester, Henwick Grove, Worcester WR2 6AJ. Publishes pollen counts and forecasts during the hay fever season.

Professional organisations

NATIONAL ASTHMA AND RESPIRATORY TRAINING CENTRE

National Respiratory
Training Centre
The Athenaeum
10 Church Street
Warwick
CV34 4AB
Tel: +44 (0) 1926 493313
Email: enquiries@nartc.org.uk

Provides accredited education and training in respiratory and allergic disease for health professionals in the UK and USA.

EUROPEAN FEDERATION OF ASTHMA AND ALLERGY ASSOCIATIONS

http://www.efanet.org

The official website for the European Federation of Asthma & Allergy Associations whose mission is to promote better health for people with asthma and allergy throughout Europe.

EUROPEAN ACADEMY OF ALLERGOLOGY AND CLINICAL IMMUNOLOGY (EAACI)
EAACI Executive Office
PO Box 24140
SE-104 51
Stockholm
Sweden

http://www.eaaci.org

Aims to promote basic and clinical research by collecting, assessing and disseminating scientific information. More than 2500 active members, works closely with 39 National Societies.

GENERAL PRACTICE AIRWAYS GROUP (UK)
8th Floor
Edgbaston House
3 Duchess Place
Edgbaston
Birmingham
B16 8NH
Tel: 0121 454 8219
Fax: 0121 454 1190

http://www.gpiag-asthma.org/

Represents primary care perspectives in respiratory medicine and aims to raise standards of care by research, innovation and dissemination of best practice. Offers a variety of 'opinion' sheets (formerly called factsheets) for GPs, primary care nurses and other allied healthcare professionals, and produces the quarterly Primary Care Respiratory Journal.

GENERAL PRACTITIONERS' ASTHMA GROUP (AUSTRALIA)
http://www.nationalasthma.org.au/resources/gpag/gpag.html

General Practitioners' Asthma Group (GPAG), part of the Australian National Asthma Council, acting as an advisory panel to the National Asthma Campaign on general practice issues, and developing and implementing various general practice initiatives for the NAC.

AMERICAN ACADEMY OF ALLERGY, ASTHMA AND IMMUNOLOGY
611 East Wells Street
Milwaukee, WI 53202
Tel: (414) 272-6071
Patient Information and Physician Referral Line: 1-800-822-2762
Email: info@aaaai.org

http://www.aaaai.org/

Latest allergy news and information for professionals, patients and the media, including pollen counts.

NATIONAL INSTITUTE OF ALLERGY AND INFECTIOUS DISEASES (NIAID) (USA)

NIAID
Building 31
Room 7A-50
31 Center Drive
MSC 2520
Bethesda
MD 20892-2520

http://www.niaid.nih.gov/default.htm

Support for scientists conducting research aimed at developing better ways to diagnose, treat and prevent the many infectious, immunologic and allergic diseases that afflict people worldwide. Offers free factsheets and brochures to download.

BRITISH SOCIETY FOR ALLERGY AND CLINICAL IMMUNOLOGY

PO Box 35649
London SE9 1WA
Tel: 020 8859 6118

http://www.bsaci.org

Professional association of clinical allergists and allergy researchers in UK. Maintains a list of National Health Service allergy clinics which is available to General Practitioners and health professionals wishing to refer patients.

BRITISH DIETETIC ASSOCIATION

7th Floor, Elizabeth House
22 Suffolk St, Queensway
Birmingham B1 1LS
Tel: 0121 643 5483
Fax: 0121 633 4399

http://www.bda.uk.com/

Association of dietitians, but may also provide information on local dietitians and offer diet information resources.

BRITISH ASSOCIATION OF DERMATOLOGISTS

http://www.skinhealth.co.uk

Professional association of skin specialists. Website has many useful leaflets on skin disease, including eczema and urticaria, as well as contact details for patient organisations.

Research, guidelines and best practice

http://bmj.com/cgi/collection/allergy

Collected resources on allergy.

http://intl.elsevierhealth.com/allergy/journals.cfm

Home site of various medical journals on allergy and related topics, including
– Asthma Magazine
– Immunology and Allergy Clinics
– Journal of Allergy and Clinical Immunology
– Skin and Allergy News
– Year Book of Allergy and Immunology.

www.blackwellmunksgaard.com/allergy

European Journal of Allergy and Clinical Immunology.

www.blackwellpublishing.com.cea

Clinical and Experimental Allergy.

http://allergy.edoc.com/

Annals of Asthma, Allergy & Immunology, official publication of the American College of Allergy, Asthma, & Immunology.

http://www.gpiag-asthma.org/Journal/JIndex.htm

Primary Care Respiratory Journal (formerly Asthma in General Practice), the official journal of the General Practice Airways Group (GPIAG) and the International Primary Care Respiratory Group (IPCRG).

http://www.doh.gov.uk/cmo/cmo989.htm

Chief Medical Officer's guidance on peanut allergy.

http://www.brit-thoracic.org.uk/sign/index.htm

British Thoracic Society – SIGN Guidelines on Asthma Management, 2003.

http://cebm.jr2.ox.ac.uk/

UK Centre for Evidence Based Medicine

Allergen extract manufacturers

ALK-ABELLO
http://www.alk-abello.com/

ALLERGOPHARMA
http://www.allergopharma.com/

DIAGENICS
(UK distributors for Allergopharma)
Diagenics Ltd
41 Barton Road
Bletchley
Milton Keynes MK2 3HU

http://www.diagenics.co.uk

STALLERGENES SA
6 rue Alexis de Tocqueville
92183 Anthony
France

HOLLISTER STIER
Hollister Stier Laboratories LLC
PO Box 3145
Spokane WA
USA

BIODIAGNOSTICS
(UK distributor for Stallergenes and Hollister Stier)
Biodiagnostics
Upton Industrial Estate
Rectory Road
Upton upon Severn
Worcs WR8 0LX
Email: enquiries@biodiagnostics.co.uk

Nut-free products

www.itsnutfree.com
www.sainsburys.co.uk

FURTHER READING

CHAPTER 1: ALLERGY AND ALLERGENS

Epidemiology and risk factors for allergy

Barraclough R et al. 2002 Apparent but not real increase in asthma prevalence in the 1990s. Eur. Respir. J. 20:826–33.

Custovic A, Hallam CL, Simpson BM, Craven M, Simpson A, Woodcock A 2001 Decreased prevalence of sensitisation to cats with high exposure to cat allergen. J. Allergy Clin. Immunol. 108:537–9.

Dharmage S et al. 2002 Mouldy houses influence symptoms of asthma among atopic individuals. Clin. Exp. Allergy 32:714–20.

Gruber C et al. 2001 Do early childhood immunisations influence the development of atopy and do they cause allergic reactions? Paed. Allergy Immunol. 12:296–311.

Guerra S et al. 2002 Rhinitis as an independent risk factor for adult-onset asthma. J. Allergy Clin. Immunol. 109:419–25.

Heinrich J et al. 2002 Trends on prevalence of atopic diseases and allergic sensitisation in children in Eastern Germany. Eur. Respir. J. 19:1040–6.

Illi S, von Mutius E, Lau S et al. 2001 The pattern of atopic sensitisation is associated with the development of asthma in childhood. J. Allergy Clin. Immunol. 108:709–14.

Kilpilainen M et al. 2001 Home dampness, current allergic diseases and respiratory infections among young adults. Thorax 56:462–7.

Koenig JQ 1999 Air pollution and asthma. J. Allergy Clin. Immunol. 104:717–22.

Simpson BM et al. 2001 NAC Manchester Asthma and Allergy Study: risk factors for asthma and allergic disorders. Clin. Exp. Allergy 31:391–9.

Strannegaard O, Strannegaard IL 2001 The causes of the increasing prevalence of allergy: is allergy a microbial deprivation disorder? Allergy 56:91–102.

von Ehrenstein OS et al. 2000 Reduced risk of hay fever and asthma among children of farmers. Clin. Exp. Allergy 30:187–93.

Wahn U, Lau S, Bergmann R et al. 1997 Indoor allergen exposure is a risk factor for sensitisation during the first three years of life. J. Allergy Clin. Immunol. 99:763–9.

Williamson IJ, Martin CJ, McGill G, Monie RDH, Fennerty AG 1997 Damp housing and asthma: a case control study. Thorax 52:229–34.

Wood RA, Chapman MD, Adkinson NF, Eggleston PA 1989 The effect of cat removal on allergen content in household dust samples. J. Allergy Clin. Immunol. 83:730–4.

Zock JP et al. 2002 Housing characteristics, reported mold exposure, and asthma in the European Community Respiratory Health Survey. J. Allergy Clin. Immunol. 110:285–92.

Immunotherapy

Abramson M, Puy R, Weiner J 1999 Immunotherapy in asthma: an updated systematic review. Allergy 54:1022–41.

Asero R 1998 Effects of birch pollen-specific immunotherapy on apple allergy in birch pollen-hypersensitive patients. Clin. Exp. Allergy 28:1368–73.

Durham SR, Walker SM, Varga EM et al. 1999 Long-term clinical efficacy of grass pollen immunotherapy. N. Engl. J. Med 341:468–75.

Malling HJ, Abreu-Nogueira J, Alvarez-Cuesta E et al. 1998 Local immunotherapy (position paper). Allergy 53:933–44.

Varney VA, Edwards J, Tabbah K, Brewster H, Mavroleon G, Frew AJ 1997 Clinical efficacy of specific immunotherapy to cat dander: a double blind placebo controlled trial. Clin. Exp. Allergy 27:860–7.

CHAPTER 2: ASTHMA

American Thoracic Society 1962 Definitions and classifications of chronic bronchitis, asthma and pulmonary emphysema. Am. Rev. Respir. Dis. 85:762–8.

Belvisi M 1996 Beta-blocker-induced asthma: a role for sensory nerve hyperresponsiveness. Clin. Exp. Allergy 26:1343–6.

British Thoracic Society/ Scottish Intercollegiate Guidelines Network 2003 British guidelines on the management of asthma. Thorax 58(S1) i1–i93

http://www.brit-thoracic.org.uk/sign/index.htm

http://www.sign.ac.uk/guidelines/

Chung KF, Godard P 2000 Difficult therapy-resistant asthma. Eur. Respir. Rev. 10(69).

Cowan S, Morin S, Ernst P 1998 Bisphosphonates and glucocorticoid-induced osteoporosis: implication for patients with respiratory diseases. Thorax 53:331–2.

Katz PP et al. 2002 Perceived control of asthma and quality of life among adults with asthma. Ann. Allergy Asthma Immunol. 89:251–8.

Reed CE 1999 The natural history of asthma in adults: the problem of irreversibility. J. Allergy Clin. Immunol. 103:539–47.

Ringsberg KC, Akerlind I 1999 Presence of hyperventilation in patients with asthma-like symptoms but negative asthma test responses: provocation with voluntary hyperventilation and mental stress. J. Allergy Clin. Immunol. 103:601–8.

Schatz M et al. 1999 The pharmacotherapy of asthma during pregnancy: current recommendations and future research. J. Allergy Clin. Immunol. 103(2 pt 2):S329–S376.

Schermer TR et al. 2002 Randomised controlled economic evaluation of asthma self-management in primary health care. Am. J. Respir. Crit. Care Med. 166:1062–72.

Weiner P et al. 1998 Characteristics of asthma in the elderly. Eur. Respir. J. 12:564–8.

CHAPTER 3: RHINITIS

AAAAI, ACAAI, JCAAI Joint Task Force 1998 Parameters for the diagnosis and management of sinusitis. J. Allergy Clin. Immunol. 102(6 pt 2):S107–S144.

Meltzer EO et al. 2000 Concomitant montelukast and loratadine as treatment for seasonal allergic rhinitis. A randomised placebo-controlled clinical trial. J. Allergy Clin. Immunol. 105:917–22.

Monteseirin J et al. 2001 Honeymoon rhinitis. Allergy 56: 353–4.

van Cauwenberge P, Bachert C, Passalacqua G et al. 2000 Consensus statement on the treatment of allergic rhinitis. Allergy 55:116–34.

CHAPTER 6: ANAPHYLAXIS

Bock SA et al. 2001 Fatalities due to anaphylactic reactions to foods. J. Allergy Clin. Immunol. 107:191–3.

Kemp S, Lockey RF 2002 Anaphylaxis: a review of causes and mechanisms. J. Allergy Clin. Immunol. 110:341–8.

Latex allergy

2002 Natural rubber latex sensitivity. J. Allergy Clin. Immunol. 110:S1–S140.

Drug allergy

Novalbos A et al. 2001 Lack of allergic cross-reactivity to cephalosporins among patients allergic to penicillins. Clin. Exp. Allergy 31:438–43.

Romano A et al. 2000 Immediate allergic reactions to cephalosporins: cross-reactivity and selective responses. J. Allergy Clin. Immunol. 106:1177–83.

Szczeklik A, Nizankowska E, Duplaga M 2000 Natural history of aspirin-induced asthma. Eur. Respir. J. 16:432–6.

Insect venom

Golden DBK et al. 1997 Natural history of hymenoptera venom sensitivity in adults. J. Allergy Clin. Immunol. 100:760–6.

Golden DBK, Kagey-Sobotka A, Lichtenstein LM 2000 Survey of patients after discontinuing venom immunotherapy. J. Allergy Clin. Immunol. 105:385–90.

Oude Elberink JNG et al. 2002 Venom immunotherapy improves health-related quality of life in patients allergic to yellow jacket venom. J. Allergy Clin. Immunol. 110:174–82.

CHAPTER 7: ANGIOEDEMA AND URTICARIA

Borges MS, Capriles-Hulett A, Caballero-Fonseca F, Perez CR 2001 Tolerability to new COX-2 inhibitors in NSAID-sensitive patients with cutaneous reactions. Ann. Allergy Asthma Immunol. 87:201–4.

Erbagci Z 2002 The leukotriene receptor antagonist montelukast in the treatment of chronic idiopathic urticaria: a single-blind placebo-controlled, crossover study. J. Allergy Clin. Immunol. 110:484–8.

Irani C et al. 2001 Chronic urticaria/angioedema and Graves' disease: coexistence of two anti-receptor antibody-mediated diseases. J. Allergy Clin. Immunol. 108:874.

Leznoff A et al. 1989 Syndrome of idiopathic chronic urticaria and angioedema with thyroid autoimmunity: a study of 90 patients. J. Allergy Clin. Immunol. 84:66–71.

Niinimäki A et al. 1998 Contact urticaria from protein hydrolysates in hair conditioners. Allergy 53:1078–82.

Perez C et al. 2001 Pretreatment with montelukast blocks NSAID-induced urticaria and angioedema. J. Allergy Clin. Immunol. 108:1060.

Tong LJ, Balakrishnan G, Kochan J, Kinet JP, Kaplan AP 1997 Assessment of autoimmunity in patients with chronic urticaria. J. Allergy Clin. Immunol. 99:461–5.

Zuberbier T et al. 2000 Anti-FceR1alpha serum autoantibodies in different types of urticaria. Allergy 55:951–4.

Reimers A et al. 2002 Zafirlukast has no beneficial effects in the treatment of chronic urticaria. Clin. Exp. Allergy 32:1763–8.

CHAPTER 8: ECZEMA

Hanifin J, Rajka G 1980 Diagnostic features of atopic dermatitis. Acta Dermatol.Venereol.(Stockh) 92:44–7.

Isolauri E et al. 2000 Probiotics in the management of atopic eczema. Clin. Exp. Allergy 30:1604–10.

Lintu P et al. 2001 Systemic ketoconazole is an effective treatment of atopic dermatitis with IgE-mediated sensitivity to yeast. Allergy 56:512–7.

Worm M et al. 2000 Clinical relevance of food additives in adult patients with atopic dermatitis. Clin. Exp. Allergy 30:407–14.

CHAPTER 9: FOOD ALLERGY

Arshad SH, Gant C 2001 Allergy to nuts: how much of a problem really is this? Clin. Exp. Allergy 31:5–7.

Beyer K et al. 2001 Effects of cooking methods on peanut allergenicity. J. Allergy Clin. Immunol. 107:1077–81.

Grundy J et al. 2002 Rising prevalence of allergy to peanut in children: data from two sequential cohorts. J. Allergy Clin. Immunol. 110:784–9.

Kanny G et al. 2001 No correlation between wine intolerance and histamine content of wine. J. Allergy Clin. Immunol. 107:375–8.

Kelso JM 2000 Pollen-food allergy syndrome. Clin. Exp. Allergy 30:905–7.

Mäkinen-Kiljunen S 1994 Banana allergy in patients with immediate-type hypersensitivity to natural rubber latex: characterisation of cross-reacting antibodies and allergens. J. Allergy Clin. Immunol. 93:990–6.

Maleki SJ et al. 2000 The effects of roasting on the allergenic properties of peanut proteins. J. Allergy Clin. Immunol. 106:763–8.

Matsuse H et al. 2001 Screening for acetaldehyde dehydrogenase 2 genotype in alcohol-induced asthma by using the ethanol patch test. J. Allergy Clin. Immunol. 108:715–9.

Ortolani C et al. 1999 Controversial aspects of adverse reactions to food. EAACI position paper. Allergy 54:27–45.

Sampson HA 1999 Food Allergy. Part 1: Immunopathogenesis and Clinical Disorders. J. Allergy Clin. Immunol. 103:717–28.

Sampson HA 1999 Food Allergy. Part 2: Diagnosis and Management. J. Allergy Clin. Immunol. 103:981–9.

Sanchez-Monge R et al. 2000 Class I chitinases, the panallergens responsible for the latex-fruit syndrome, are induced by ethylene treatment and inactivated by heating. J. Allergy Clin. Immunol. 106:190–5.

Sicherer SH et al. 1999 Self-reported allergic reactions to peanut on commercial airliners. J. Allergy Clin. Immunol. 104:186–9.

Sicherer SH, Sampson HA, Burks AW 2000 Peanut and soy allergy: a clinical and therapeutic dilemma. Allergy 55:515–21.

Taylor SL, Hefle SL 2001 Will genetically modified foods be allergenic? J. Allergy Clin. Immunol. 107:765–71.

Tauber SS, Brown RL, Haapanen LAD 1997 Allergenicity of gourmet nut oils

processed by different methods. J. Allergy Clin. Immunol. 99:502–7.

Woessner KM, Simon RA, Stevenson DD 1999 Monosodium glutamate sensitivity in asthma. J. Allergy Clin. Immunol. 104:305–10.

Woods RK et al. 1998 The effects of monosodium glutamate in adults with asthma who perceive themselves to be monosodium glutamate intolerant. J. Allergy Clin. Immunol. 101:762–71.

CHAPTER 10: OCCUPATIONAL ALLERGIES

Barker RD, van Tongeren MJ, Harris JM, Gardiner K, Venables KM, Newman-Taylor AJ 1998 Risk factors for sensitisation and respiratory symptoms among workers exposed to acid anhydrides: a cohort study. Occup. Environ. Med. 55:684–91.

Blanco Carmona JG et al. 1992 Occupational asthma in the confectionery industry caused by sensitivity to egg. Allergy 47:190–1.

Bush RK, Wood RA, Eggleston PA 1998 Laboratory animal allergy. J. Allergy Clin. Immunol. 102:99–112.

Estlander T et al. 1996 Occupational conjunctivitis associated with type IV allergy to methacrylates. Allergy 51:56–9.

Gannon PFG et al. 1995 Occupational asthma due to glutaraldehyde and formaldehyde in endoscopy and x-ray departments. Thorax 50:156–9.

Malo JL, Chan-Yeung M 2001 Occupational asthma. J. Allergy Clin. Immunol. 108:315–28.

Thickett KM et al. 2002 Occupational asthma caused by chloramines in indoor swimming pool air. Eur. Respir. J. 19:827–32.

Vandenplas O et al. 2001 Occupational asthma in symptomatic workers exposed to natural rubber latex: evaluation of diagnostic procedures. J. Allergy Clin. Immunol. 107:543–7.

CHAPTER 11: ALLERGIES IN CHILDHOOD

Eggesbo M et al. 2001 The prevalence of allergy to egg: a population-based study in young children. Allergy 56:403–11.

Figueroa-Munoz JI et al. 2001 Association between obesity and asthma in 4–11 year old children. Thorax 56:133–7.

Khakoo GA, Lack G 2000 Guidelines for measles vaccination in egg-allergic patients. Clin. Exp. Allergy 30:288–92.

Vickers DW, Maynard L, Ewan PW 1997 Management of children with potential anaphylactic reactions in the community: a training package and proposal for good practice. Clin. Exp. Allergy 27:898–903.

CHAPTER 12: COMPLEMENTARY THERAPY AND ALLERGIES

AAAAI Board of Directors 1999 Position statement: idiopathic environmental intolerances. J. Allergy Clin. Immunol. 103:36–40.

de Lorenzo F, Xiao H, Mukherjee M et al. 1998 Chronic fatigue syndrome: physical and cardiovascular deconditioning. Q. J. Med. 91:475–81.

Huntley A, White AR, Ernst E 2002 Relaxation therapies for asthma. Thorax 57:127–31.

Lewith GT, Holgate ST 1999 Why integration of complementary and orthodox medicine is so important. Asthma Journal 4:8–9.

Martin J et al. 2002 Efficacy of acupuncture in asthma: systematic review and meta-analysis of published data from 11 randomised controlled trials. Eur. Respir. J. 20:846–52.

Reilly DT, Taylor MA, McSharry C, Aitchison T 1986 Is homeopathy a placebo response? Controlled trial of homeopathic potency with pollen in hay fever as a model. Lancet ii:881–6.

Semizzi M et al. 2002 A double-blind, placebo-controlled study on the diagnostic accuracy of an electrodermal test in allergic subjects. Clin. Exp. Allergy 32:928–32.

Zimens I, Tashkin DP 2000 Alternative medicine for allergy and asthma. J. Allergy Clin. Immunol. 106:603–14.

LIST OF PATIENT QUESTIONS

INDEX

Note: Page numbers in **bold** refer to figures and tables.
The word *vs* indicates a comparison in the text.
Milk refers to cow's milk unless otherwise stated.

Since the major subject of this text is 'allergy,' entries have been kept to a minimum under this keyword; readers are advised to seek more specific index entries.
Abbreviations used in this index include:
LTRA - Leukotriene receptor antagonist
MSG - Monosodium glutamate
NSAIDs - Non-steroidal anti-inflammatory drugs

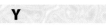